She Became
Mighty in Battle

She Became Mighty in Battle

The Face of Breast Cancer

Rebecca Johnson

To order additional copies of this book, contact:
Xlibris
844-714-8691
www.Xlibris.com
Orders@Xlibris.com
827976

CONTENTS

This is dedicated to all the fast-track women who put family and career first and probably worry about themselves less than they should. We are the women who drive that minivan around town like we are on a NASCAR track, dropping kids to various sports, attempting to move up the ladder at work by making ourselves marketable, and being the best wife we can possibly be. Sometimes tragedy comes out of left field and knocks us down a few pegs. When it happens, we are flooded with emotions. The sadness, denial, bravery, and anger roll in like a hurricane and determine our progress in moving forward. I know this all too well when I received my stage 3C breast cancer diagnosis. This whole thing stopped me in my tracks and made me reevaluate myself. I am forty-three years old, possibly facing death and leaving everything I love behind. The worst thing I had ever faced was a traditional gallbladder removal, and now this. Now I am facing the worst-case scenario and trying to put my life into perspective. What is important? I have always heard the phrase "Don't sweat the small stuff." So what is the "small stuff" in my life? My purpose for putting my journey out there is part self-reflection and a reminder to me of the struggle and also a chance to help families going through this same process. I learned so much through this journey and think it is important to know other people's successful journeys to help them battle through the bad days. I hope that looking at the real face of cancer, this book brings positivity and humor to push forward.

(Our family several months before my diagnosis at Disney
World. Left to Right TJ, Morgan, Madison, Becky)

Chapter 1

A Northeaster Took the Wind Out of My Sails

Growing up on the Eastern Shore of Virginia, I have seen my share of storms. This included northeasters, hurricanes, flooding, and even an occasional tornado, but the storms that hit my life in March of 2018 came out of left field and changed me and my family forever. My life was seemingly normal. I was a public school teacher who specialized in gifted education. My next step in my career was moving up in administration, but I just could not take that next step out of fear of moving out of my comfort zone. I was constantly having big, scary thoughts that were occupying space in my head. Would I be able to survive the cut-throat life of building administration? Could I handle the stress of running a building or program? I was constantly beating myself up over what-ifs to the point of searching out therapy. Little did I know that a storm was brewing inside of me that would change everything in this game of life.

My own health was relatively good and normal. The year prior, I had to have a gallbladder surgery that may or may not have been stress related. That was a big, monumental thing in my life. According to everyone I talked to, just about everyone had a gallbladder removal, and I was simply joining the Wonky Gallbladder Club. I felt good. I tried to make it to the local YMCA for a spin class or time on the elliptical.

I may not have been a picture of ideal fitness, but I cared enough about myself not to shop in the local Walmart in ratty pajamas and scruffy slippers like some women in town. I am married to a wonderful, caring, loving, and smart man, TJ, for fifteen years. Through our marriage, we brought two girls into the world: Madison, who had recently turned fourteen, and Morgan, who was eleven at the time of my diagnosis. I had everything I could ever need and want but didn't really realize all I had.

I had experiences with cancer. This was not my first rodeo with it since about twelve years ago. My mother was diagnosed with endometrium cancer. Mom went through six chemotherapies and over twenty radiations. I watched her pain and trials. Immediately afterward, a family friend went through liver cancer. The difference was even though both ladies were older, they had different journeys. My mother was a survivor, and our family friend went into hospice care and passed away. Seeing this was so hard and hit my mother in ways that seemed to resemble survivor's guilt. I also had a workmate and friend who was my age that was diagnosed with cancer shortly before me. Her cancer journey was short as she passed shortly after her diagnosis. My maternal grandmother had liver cancer, and my paternal grandfather had prostate cancer. Cancer was a part of my life. I was no stranger to it happening . . . to people around me, but not me! The storm of cancer was brewing inside me, but life was going on, and I was busy stressing about everything else.

I made sure to get my checkups. I made the time to get my yearly physical, mammograms, and even a dental cleaning every six months. As a mom and wife, I was the chief medical appointment organizer for everyone in the family. The news was always good, and I went on my merry way with my appointment card for the next appointment.

Then it happened. I never saw it coming.

The March morning started like every other one. It was a Monday, and I woke up dreading the morning craziness of an elementary school. The weather had been very unpredictable. There had been multiple northeasters, and the wind and rain had already put a dark cloud on this Monday. I got out of bed and talked myself out of calling in sick. TJ and I have a morning routine that continues to this day. We get up and walk our two dogs, and then he fixes coffee, and I wake up our daughters. This morning, our daily jaunt would include wind and rain. Balancing the dog who was feeling frisky because of the wind was a struggle. The wind picked up and blew open my jean jacket that I threw over my pajamas. I took my right hand to pull the jacket closed, and it happened. There was a lump in my left armpit. I had never felt it before. It was about two fingertips across and hard. What the heck is that? Was it there last night when I took my shower? I think I would have felt it because it was so large.

I came in the house, stunned. What was this thing growing on me? TJ picked up on my confusion immediately. My initial reaction was to ask him to feel it. Of course, he made some jokes about feeling my breasts so early in the morning and having to get to work on time. When he noticed the look of fear and confusion on my face, his mood got serious. He felt it, stepped back, and felt it again. Then he gave me a flurry of questions: Did you feel this before today? Does it hurt? Did you feel it in the shower before? What do you think it is? What are you going to do?

I stood there in our kitchen, confused. What do I do now? TJ's response was to go to the doctor. Uhhhh . . . doctor's offices are filled with people who have germs. Doesn't he realize that the killer flu is going around? The absolute last thing I need is to get the flu. I have spent this whole school year avoiding it, and now I am walking into the lion's den of germs. I had gone through a previous family care physician who basically treated me like a high-maintenance complainer. On top of that, she took every opportunity to fat-shame me. According to my BMI, I was obese. In my delusional mind, I was just curvy, but in truth, I was probably a biscuit away from two hundred pounds.

TJ said that I needed to quit my bitching and just go.

Finally, after some discussion, I agreed to head out to work and make the call to the doctor. I made every excuse in the world to not call the medical center for an appointment, but I finally decided that if it would shut my husband up, then I would just go ahead and do it.

What is the worst they could possibly say? After I hung up the phone with the medical center, I pouted for a while about missing a half day of work. I would so much rather use my sick leave for mental health days than the actual possibility of being sick. The year prior, I had used some leave because of a gallbladder that decided that it no longer wanted to be in my presence. It seems that since turning forty, the "check engine" light of my body keeps turning on.

The entire day, I kept putting my hand on the lump. I figured that as quick as it appeared, it may disappear as well. I even thought that my luck would be that by the time I arrive at my appointment, it would probably be gone. All day and all night, I continued to check if that bump, lump, or whatever it was, was still there. I had all kinds of solutions in my head of why it was there. Maybe it is just a viral infection because don't those types of infections get in the lymph nodes? Or maybe it is a huge pimple that is trapped under the skin. It could be a razor bump since I do religiously shave my armpits (but why is it under the skin?). I had many questions and really dreaded the possibilities of getting the answers.

I had never been a sickly person, so the idea of receiving bad medical news was something that I just did not expect. My biggest worry at this time was the doctor sending me on my merry way with a disapproving glare of wasting his or her time. My doctor at this medical center was always very condescending in her tone to me. Her bedside manner was very much lacking, and it made me question myself whenever I had an issue. When I started to have issues with the gallbladder the prior year, she basically chastised me for making an appointment. About a week later, I was at the emergency room at the local hospital at two in the morning, thinking that I was having a heart attack. Luckily, that morning, I had an ER doctor who had seen these symptoms before with someone with a failing gallbladder. My family doctor had let me down in the past, and luckily, since it was a horrible flu season, she was totally booked. I was grateful that there was an appointment to see the nurse practitioner. My ultimate plan was to go in quick and go back to work before anyone noticed.

Chapter 2

Queen of Denial

The medical center that I go to is an odd little place. It is full of mismatched décor. After a recent hospital takeover, the corporation tried to "remodel" all their medical center branches. Even with new paint, new chairs, and a fancy television on the wall that played medical infomercials, it still felt weird, cold, and unwelcoming. Another thing that was irritating me was that the waiting room was filled with sick people. The flu was going through our community like an out-of-control freight train. Being someone who works in the schools, I knew that my day of catching the influenza was becoming more and more of a reality. What was even more frustrating was that even though I had a flu shot, I have willingly put myself in the line of fire with all these sick people looking like extras from a zombie movie.

After getting all the basics of paying a co-payment and showing my insurance card, I was called back for weight and blood pressure. My blood pressure was good, and I was still fat according to the scale. My main thought was that if this person fat-shames me, then out the door I go!

Everything was going well, and it was all smiles and cordial comments. The nurse practitioner came in, and she was far more pleasant than the doctor I normally see. I figured that since I was there, I should go ahead and tell her about how my left arm randomly goes numb as well and how it is happening more and more each day. We finally got down to the business of the lump. She felt it. She got a weird look on her face. Then the questions started. "When did this appear? Does it seem to get larger each day or stay the same? Does it hurt when touched? Can you put your arm down comfortably?"

Wait, what? Is this actually something I should worry about? I couldn't get the words out of my mouth because the physician's assistant quickly exited the room to return with more people. The next thing I realized was that lots of people were coming into the room to feel this lump in my armpit. I knew that I felt gross as I was now sweating because I was nervous. Could it be that something was actually wrong with me?

The PA was very quick to send me to the blood workstation to have some labs completed. Little did I know that she was on the phone with the local hospital which housed the mammogram machines. By the time I was on my way out the door, she had printed out notes of directions for the next day. This included going to the local hospital for a mammogram and ultrasound. I tried to explain that I had a mammogram recently (as I was trying to do the math in my head) and everything was just fine. I wanted to just yell that we shouldn't overreact. I was sticking with this was probably a lymph node gone rogue. I left the office with a feeling of dread or maybe a feeling of amazement because every time I thought something was wrong with me, it was dismissed. Now I think it is nothing and everyone is freaking out.

No sooner had I gotten in the car than my phone rang, and it was TJ. Now he had a lot of questions. He could probably hear the confusion in my voice. How could this be happening? Is there something really wrong, or is just everyone overreacting? One thing I did notice was that the demeanor of everyone in that office changed. It started as friendly and excited to see me and ended with strict rules of not missing the follow-up appointments. I could feel the tension, or maybe it was pity and worry in the air. I just sat in the parking lot, talking to TJ. He was trying to cover up his worry, but I could hear it in his voice. This could be serious. He decided that the next day, he would go with me to the appointment at the hospital.

I went back to work, all along thinking about what tomorrow would bring and what I have already experienced today. Could it be the C word? There is no way! Breast cancer doesn't run in my family. All day, my thoughts ran wild with the what-ifs of this situation. I even felt the lump every five minutes to see if it was still there. It was. As the day went on, I started Googling on the computer and going to WebMD. That basically told me that I may or may not be dying. I also went to all the teachers at work that I am close to and got them to feel the lump. Of course, in my mind, it was a rouge lymph node. I had recently had a mammogram, and it was fine. It was done about a year prior, and I was called back for an ultrasound because of dense breast tissue. After it was all done, I was released with a clean bill of health. So why am I worried? I have other things to take care of. My oldest daughter is turning fourteen, and we have a party planned this weekend at Great Wolf Lodge, an indoor water park with her friends and younger sister. I have to be on mom duty this upcoming weekend, so I need to get these appointments behind me and move forward.

I worked the next day in the morning and then would meet my husband at the hospital where they do mammograms. The physician's assistant also ordered an ultrasound. All morning at work, I would teach my classes and rush back to my office to check the patient portal to see if the results of my blood work had been posted. It was posted, and of course, I had no clue what it meant. My husband at the time was the Dean of Workforce at our local community college. Employed at the college was a doctor who ran the nursing program. If I cannot figure out what this blood work means, then I'm sure the head of the nursing program could make some sense of it. I e-mailed it to my husband, TJ, with strict directions to show it to the doctor. Of course, the doctor looked at it and said, "I need more information."

Uhhhh, can someone just tell me everything is okay?

Finally, the time arrived for me to embark to the hospital for the appointment. TJ was waiting for me in the hospital parking lot, and we walked in together. The thing about living in a small town is that gossip runs rampant. Being in the hospital waiting room will start all kinds of small-town rumors. What will the rumors be? Maybe that I am pregnant? Got cancer? Bleeding out the butt? My husband is getting a vasectomy? There are so many possibilities.

One thing that struck me with this experience was that I was offered two different types of mammograms. I could have a regular mammogram or a 3D mammogram. The catch was that the 3D cost more, and the cost may not be completely covered by my health insurance. I am fortunate to have great insurance, and why not continue my high-maintenance ways and get the best mammogram. All the while, the thought kept lingering about this mammogram thing. What if I didn't have the money or the good insurance coverage? Would I have taken a lower level of treatment? That stayed on my mind and made me mad. Why, as women, do we have to make a choice based on money? Shouldn't we always get the best treatment?

I didn't have to ponder this for long because the technician called me back in for the 3D mammogram. I went in for this unenjoyable experience. The technician took all kinds of pictures, but I was not smiling. I just wanted to get this over with and get this whole experience behind me. Not so fast, this event is not over yet. The technician introduced me to the ultrasound technician who would take me to the ultrasound room. So I basically got undressed, dressed, so I could get undressed again. The ultrasound tech was very young, and I was checking to see if I taught her in elementary school. Luckily, I did not teach her. The last thing I needed was one of my former fourth graders feeling on my boobs. She took a lot of pictures, none of which I smiled for. I was waiting for the okay to put my top back on and go home. All of a sudden, the tech said, "I sent the pictures to Dr. William, and he would like to talk to you." I looked at her a bit confused and said, "Why?" Before she could respond, a small stature man entered the room and introduced himself as Dr. William. After going through the introductions, he started to use the ultrasound machine himself. He kept looking at various spots from my armpit to my lower left breast. He was also taking more pictures of the same spots that the tech had already taken. He asked if anyone was with me today.

"Yes, my husband is in the waiting room."

The technician quickly exited the room and reappeared in minutes, with TJ in tow. Everyone looked worried, and I was waiting to put my shirt back on. Once we got settled and I put my shirt on, Dr. William explained that I had two places of concern: the lump in my armpit and the lump deep in the bottom of my left breast. The second lump showed up on the mammogram and was in a spot that could not be felt but was large enough to show up in 3D.

Dr. William went on about how he wanted to do a biopsy on the original lump in my armpit. When is this going to happen? Just in two days. Really? I need time to think about this! The doctor was quick to tell me that this is something we don't wait for, and his first available appointment was on Friday. Today was Wednesday, and I had plans for the weekend.

Dr. William said that a biopsy was easy. He would cut open the lump and take a piece to biopsy. Could I drive myself home? Yes, of course. Could I still go away for the weekend? Yes, of course. Can I get the spot wet since we are going to an indoor water park this weekend? What does this all mean? Is this serious? I was full of questions, and I wasn't hearing that everything was fine. I was just getting the answer of no definite answer until the biopsy results return. I wanted answers now! I don't want to wait however long the lab would take to process the biopsy.

Within the two days of waiting for my biopsy appointment, I did all the things that a patient should not do. I was Googling and watching biopsy videos. These were the things one should not do when facing an impending biopsy procedure. I went to work, but my mind was on this procedure. Dr. William said it was easy. Maybe easy for him, but will it be easy for me?

The morning arrived, and my mother convinced me that she should drive me over to the hospital. She was on high alert with this situation as she is a uterine cancer survivor. In my mind, this was going to be a big waste of time. The lab would look in that microscope and see nothing of importance. Meanwhile, I would have worry and miss work.

A nurse brought me back and started to prep all the materials and clean the targeted area. She explained everything that was going to happen, including showing me a metal ribbon that Dr. William would place in the area of the incision to mark the spot that was removed. As I looked at the metal marker, I realized it was shaped like one of those cancer ribbons. *Why am I getting one of those? I don't have cancer, or do I?* Seeing that marker made my heart drop. *Is this really happening?* I asked the nurse if she thought I had cancer. *Do they use that particular marker on cancer patients? Can I get a different one since I probably don't have cancer?* The nurse looked at me, and her face looked sad. She knew but couldn't say anything until the result came back.

Dr. William came rushing in and was ready for action. He was chipper and ready to do this since I was the first appointment of the day. As we started the process, he explained everything that was going to happen, but my mind was definitely elsewhere. I did hear him say that he would inject a numbing solution into the area that he would cut. I clearly heard that if I were to feel uncomfortable, I could request more of this numbing solution. When it comes to pain, I have no problem asking to be comfortable. The plan was to only test the area from my armpit. He said that he did not need to gain samples from the spot within my left breast.

As he started, I felt my anxiety levels rising. The numbing injection was supposed to be the worst part of this, and the process of gaining the sample was to be quick. I was in an uncomfortable position with my arm above my head and lying on my side. I was using sound as an indicator of how this process was going since I could not see because of my position. Honestly, I did not want to see what was going on. I just wanted it over. Listening to Dr. William, I was hearing noises that put me on red alert. Sounds like "Hmmmm . . . interesting . . ." Finally, I couldn't take it anymore.

"Are you done yet? You said this would be quick, and that does not seem to be the case."

I knew I took him off guard because he stopped and explained that he was having difficulty getting the sample from the lump. The numbing solution was wearing off, and the pain was starting to grow. I was officially uncomfortable and, in many words (some of which would fall under the category of obscenity), let him know it was time for another injection.

After several more injections to manage pain, a sample was finally removed. At that point, all parties involved were breathing a sigh of relief. The ribbon clip was placed at the location of removal, and I was definitely ready to exit the appointment.

"So when will I see you again for the results of this?" I asked.

"We should have the results back from the lab by Tuesday or Wednesday. My nurse will call you, and we will meet to review. Don't worry about this and enjoy your weekend away with your family. And by the way, stay off the internet and no Googling symptoms. It just gets people upset."

Chapter 3

Throwing Care to the Wolves

I spent the day of the biopsy in bed. It was physically and mentally exhausting. Every time my mind thought that there was a possibility of this being cancer, I shook away the thought. TJ continually asked me if I could handle this birthday trip to Great Wolf Lodge, a hotel and indoor water park. Of course, I could handle this, and I would. What kind of mother would I be if I bailed out of my oldest daughter's fourteenth birthday celebration? We had a large suite, and that would accommodate our daughters, Madison and Morgan; TJ; myself; and three of Madison's friends. It was going to be a great time full of waterslides, pizza, and even a giant cream puff doughnut from our town's local bakery. There was something that was lurking. It was the unknown. The emotion of what might happen.

The car ride there, I didn't hear the giggling and singing of teenage girls. My thoughts were huge and scary. What if . . . What if this is really something serious? Why did Dr. William have problems getting into this lump? All I could see in my mind's eye was the looks I received at all of these appointments. It seemed like everyone knew something, but no one wanted to come forth and tell me.

I was only about forty minutes from home, and it happened. I have always been one to believe in signs, and I got a sign that I was not expecting. It was literally a sign. A billboard on the side of the highway.

It had a picture of about five doctors in their white coats looking very official. The man in the center was none other than Dr. William. There he was, larger than life with a smile. The slogan was an advertisement for the local hospital with the phrase "Your local cancer center team." I thought I would drive off the road. My eyes teared up, and my chest felt tight. *Cancer* . . . There it was, the word that I was avoiding. Not only was the word there, but also the doctor who just did my biopsy was on a damn highway billboard. I realized that no one in the car noticed what I just did. They were still laughing and excited for fun, and I was privately freaking out.

Since we had some many children and not enough space, we had to take two vehicles. When we stopped for lunch, I asked TJ if he had seen the hospital billboard. He did not notice it but was concerned that I was concerned. I played it off and joked about seeing Dr. William on the billboard. It was important to get off this topic because the more I bring it up, the more worried I become. This was not a time to worry about me; this was time to celebrate a birthday.

We arrived, and the chaos of checking in with many excited teenagers blurred my worry. Everything was going good, and I had pushed the big scary cancer thoughts far away. I ordered and ate pizza, played skee-ball, and laughed with the kids like a mom not facing a devastating illness. Once the kids were sort of settled down, TJ and I went to our room to sleep and did exactly what Dr. William said not to do. I was on Facebook, and suddenly on my page, there was a site for women facing breast cancer diagnosis. I swear our phones listen to us! Here it was proving my crazy theory. Should I click on it? If I click on it, it will probably prove that I am just overreacting to a situation that is probably nothing. I clicked on it. There it was, story after story of women being diagnosed with breast cancer. There were women who found lumps, women who went for mammograms, cancer at every stage, and even caregivers talking about how they dealt with cancer and with losing a loved one. I didn't last a half hour. The tears were welling up, and my chest was tightening. TJ rolled over and asked if I was all right. I couldn't cover it anymore.

"What if this is bad?" I asked.

"Well, wrap your head around the fact that this could be something bad. Be prepared to deal with the possibility of cancer," he responded. "I'm here for you. We are always a team, no matter what."

I didn't sleep well that night. There were big scary thoughts, but none of them came close to the reality I was about to face. I continued this weekend with on and off thoughts of what the future would look like, along with trying to act like a super mom. Yes, I just had a biopsy, and yes, I was going down waterslides. No one except TJ had any clue what I was carrying around with me during this weekend. One of my favorite pictures was a picture of TJ and I in the lobby of Great Wolf Lodge. We were smiling and having fun on the surface, but the fear of the future was deep. It was the last picture of me with hair before treatment.

The workweek started, and it was time to wait for the results, and my mind was all over the place. I called Dr. William on Monday and Tuesday. He had received the results but needed to review them and wanted to meet with me on Wednesday at one o'clock. The beginning of the week seemed like everything was moving in slow motion. On Tuesday, I was working at a school that the principal was a friend from childhood named Jennifer. We had known each other since we were four years old in ballet class. She was in her office, working on paperwork, and knocked on the office door. "Do you have a minute? I want to talk to you before you hear town gossip."

"Yeah, girl. Get in here and close the door. Are you okay?"

"Well, I found a lump in my armpit, and the doctor sent me for a mammogram and ultrasound, and then the doctor wanted to biopsy it. I find out everything tomorrow."

Jennifer sat there with tears in her eyes. She didn't say anything for a while. We just sat there looking at each other. I didn't know what to do, so I just kept talking.

"I'm sure it will be nothing, but I am spending a lot of time at the hospital getting these different procedures, and I have already seen one person from the school board office at that hospital, and that is how the rumors start. I have been friends with you for such a long time that I would not want you to hear this as a rumor."

Jennifer got up from her seat and walked around her desk and hugged me. "No matter what you hear tomorrow, I am here for you."

I spent a long time in her office. We laughed, cried, and talked about how we were too young for this. Jennifer had her own experiences with health issues, and we were starting to wonder if there was something about turning forty that makes everything start to break down. Jennifer felt the lump and listened to the whole story. She kept telling me that everything was going to be okay, but I could see the worry in her eyes. It was the same look that I had seen all the previous week from the doctors and nurses.

Wednesday finally arrived. I had a lot of sleepless nights. Could this lump be some sort of breast cancer? It doesn't run in my family, so how did this situation occur to me? Then my mind would turn to thinking that there is no possible way that this could happen to me. TJ was going with me to find out the biopsy results. We had five days of discussing the what-ifs of this situation, but there was no way to prepare for what was going to happen.

TJ and I met in the hospital parking lot and walked in together. It was a quiet walk. I checked in, and we sat in the lobby, waiting to go back. All I could think was I was looking forward to the moment of being told that everything is okay and walking back to the car laughing about how silly we were to be worried about nothing. The nurse called us back but took us to another waiting room. TJ kept holding my hand and telling me that everything will be okay. Finally, Dr. William appeared.

"Becky, we are going to go back to a conference room and talk. I am waiting for the outreach nurse to join us."

We walked to this little room that looked like another version of a waiting room with single chairs along the walls. Dr. William was upbeat and keeping the small talk with TJ. As for me, I just wanted to get this going and go home. Finally, an older lady arrived and introduced herself as the outreach nurse for the cancer center.

"Why is she here? Do I have cancer?"

Dr. William could tell that I was in freak out mode, so he started quickly. "I received your biopsy back from the lab. Let's talk about what the results show. The left axillary biopsy results were positive. Specifically, pathology demonstrated invasive ductal carcinoma."

We spent about twenty minutes listening to Dr. William and the outreach nurse discuss the results and "pathways" of what is the course of action. I didn't hear a word that they said. I heard the words *breast cancer*, and I mentally exited. How could this be possible? I could hear TJ talking to the doctor. He was asking the questions that I should have been asking, but I could not get myself together to make a clear thought. Finally, Dr. William asked me if I was okay. The only clear sentence that I could string together was to ask if he was sure that he was looking at my file. It could not possibly be me that he was talking about. Cancer? I felt like I was falling, and there was nothing to catch myself.

The patient outreach nurse offered to take me on a tour of the cancer center. TJ had to slip away to pick up our daughters from school. This left me alone with the outreach nurse. I was not sure of the vibe I was getting from her. She was nice, but I was not focused on making pleasantries. Then she said it. It was not meant in a rude manner, but it was something that stuck with me through the entire process. She touched my hair and said, "Your hair is so beautiful. It is a shame that you will lose it, but it will come back. It will probably come back just as pretty." Everything from there on was a blur.

Chapter 4

Am I Ready for This?

I don't think that what was happening ever did sink into my brain. Some would say that I was delusional or that I was covering up my feelings. Honestly, I didn't know how to feel. I saw my own mother go through cancer treatment, but did this experience make me knowledgeable? This is when I started to learn that each person, even if they have the same type of cancer, have a different journey.

Several ladies in my community were diagnosed with breast cancer shortly before me. They had already started the process. They were the talk of the community. There was lots of talk of their age as they were around my age. In a tight-knit community, everyone jumps on being super helpful in the beginning. There is always the typical fundraiser or GoFundMe pages started. I don't want anyone to feel sorry for me. One of the things that I hate the most is someone making a sad face and pouting out their bottom lip at me with a "bless your heart" thrown in here and there. It feels very disingenuous, and I try to stay away from situations that may involve that. The more I thought about my own situation and saw what these other ladies were dealing with made me want to invert into a little bubble and not tell anyone what was going on.

I still could not wrap my mind around this. How could this happen? What is going to happen? Before I left the cancer center, I was given several appointments. The first was meeting with one of the oncologists.

The second appointment was a breast MRI. This MRI was going to be at a diagnostic center two hours away from home. I had to go this far because my hospital MRI machine did not have the software to complete this breast procedure. Little did I know that I was going to be overwhelmed with appointments. The culmination of the field trip to the cancer center was walking out to the car to meet TJ and my phone text message ring going off. It was a text from the imaging center that I normally go to, saying that I was due for my mammogram. Guess, they are a little late to the party because I am now beyond needing a mammogram. That was the thing that made this hard to process. It was not like I had avoided getting a mammogram. Quite the contrary, I was going to my scheduled appointments and was getting the green light that everything was fine. When I say that this situation blindsided me, I was not joking or exaggerating. As a matter of fact, the last mammogram I had sent me to get an ultrasound because they felt that since I had so much dense tissue in my breasts, they wanted to make sure they could see everything. Dense tissue is just a nice way of saying "you are fat and you carry a lot of fat in your boobs."

The afternoon of finding out that I officially had cancer, TJ and I talked to our children about it. This was something that I was terribly nervous about. I have worked as a public school teacher for over twenty years, and I have seen firsthand how a traumatic event can effect a child. Now the situation is how to help my own children cope during our new family tragedy. My oldest daughter, Madison, was in eighth grade and tried to always act like she was grown. She had always been an A student. School was important to her, and she is very athletic. Morgan was in the fifth grade and was definitely not as mature. She still liked to play and wear JoJo bows in her hair. She has always been a little sassy and a free spirit. I didn't want this situation to have a negative effect on either one of them. I didn't want them to worry about losing their mom, but that was a promise that I may not be able to keep. I remember getting in the car and the girls were already there. I had been crying while doing my tour of the cancer center. There was no amount of makeup that could cover that I was upset. When the girls saw me, they both stopped talking. TJ started with the "Girls, your mom and

I have some news for you." We never thought that we would have this conversation with the girls, so we were not prepared. I don't think you can even prepare for that conversation. There are probably great books and articles about how to tell your children that you have cancer, but I never took the time to reference that. There was no getting around this, and it came blurted out.

"The doctor told your mom that she has cancer, but she is going to get treatment and get better." Morgan took it at face value with an "Okay and what are we doing for dinner." Madison, on the other hand, was inquisitive. She wanted to know the hows, whats, and whys of this situation. Most of that I had no answer for. That night, we told the girls, my mother-in-law and her friend Judy, my parents, two friends I taught with, Christy Anne and Karrie, and my friend Krysten and her husband Chuck. For Krysten, the pain was deep as she had lost her mother to a battle with cancer. Because of that, she had always thrown herself into a local fundraising with Relay For Life and spent most her time involved in Relay events. Telling people who are close to you is extremely difficult. I didn't want those people to hurt because of me. When I would see the tears welling up in their eyes, I felt like I had to do or say something to make it better. I caught myself telling those people that "It would be okay" or that "I'm a tough old bird" or that "You can't get rid of me that easy." Deep down, that reassuring manner didn't exist. I was scared and not feeling like a fighter or even the slightest amount tough. I made them all swear to secrecy. I wanted to know more before I tell the masses about my diagnosis. At this moment, all I know was that I am a cancer patient, and that is where it ends. I wanted solid information such as a stage or simply if I am going to die. Some questions I would never get the answer to, and some were going to be answered in the near future.

My first appointment at the cancer center was the very next morning. It was a sleepless night of wondering what was going to happen. TJ and I lay in bed, holding hands and reminiscing of good times during our many years of marriage. He made the promise that no matter what, we were a team and going to fight this together. I was grateful to hear that, but I also remember a woman whom I worked with who had breast cancer and her husband left her during treatment. I understood that this was going to be a tough journey not just for me but also for TJ and our girls. It was a time that I silently pondered if our family would survive this.

The time arrived for the appointment. I was worried for all the normal reasons, but also because instead of seeing the regular oncologist that I would see throughout my treatment, I would see the oncologist who was going to retire within the next week. The oncologist I was to see was away at a medical conference, and apparently, my medical situation required me not to wait for the regular oncologist's return.

The retiring oncologist had been the attending doctor for so long that the infusion wing at the cancer center was named after him. I was confident that he was knowledgeable, but was he updated in the latest of cancer practices? I know in education, I enjoyed working with the younger teachers. They had new ideas and were excited about what they were doing and eager to try things in the classroom. The veteran teachers were usually the ones that complained and never tried new things (because we have always done things this way). I hope this is not the same in the medical field. Yes, I sound very ageist, but I have dealt with some stubborn old people, and I am no spring chicken myself.

The patient outreach worker was going to attend my appointment with me. I went into the doctor's small office. I could tell that he was in the process of packing up a lifetime of his career. He was kind and seemed to have a good bedside manner. Once again, he explained that he would not be my doctor but did not want to wait to review this information with me. In front of him was the paperwork from my biopsy. I did not know all the definitions and acronyms that come with breast cancer, but as he was reviewing the information, I was shaking my head in agreement as if I knew exactly what he was talking about. I pulled little things from the conversation that helped me appear to know what was going on. He was excellent at explaining everything, but the problem was that I was terrible at listening. I just wanted to know if I was going to die. It was like he read my mind, and he put his hand on mine and said, "You will make it through this. It will be tough at times, but you will be okay." That was all I needed at that moment. There were times in this process that I would reflect back on that conversation and wonder if he told all his patients that so they didn't melt down in front of him. There were times that I wondered if he lied so that I would not ugly cry through the whole appointment.

The points that did not make sense to me at the time but were important information were that my cancer was highly aggressive. My final diagnosis was that I was facing a malignant and invasive ductal carcinoma that was a grade of 3 of 3. The pathology report even put that information in all capital letters, so obviously, they meant business. It was explained that I was barely ER positive, PR negative, and Her2 positive. This sounded like another language to me, but soon it would be a language I would become fluent.

When the doctor finished, the patient outreach nurse turned to me with a list of appointments. She had scheduled a breast MRI, a bone density scan, an echocardiogram, an appointment with a surgeon for a port, and a PET scan. *How do I work and keep this going?* It seemed like my new job was being a patient.

Chapter 5

Test Dummy

The first appointment of many was probably the toughest for me as I learned to accept my diagnosis. I had to go for a breast MRI. This appointment was located at a medical center affiliated with my hospital but was located close to two hours away from home. TJ was going to go with me, and looking back, it was a good thing that I had his support that day.

I love TJ very much, but sometimes my patience runs thin with him because of my own anxiety. He seemed very comfortable talking about work, football, and where we should get breakfast before the appointment. I now think that his over chattiness was him trying to cover his nervousness. We ended up at a Pancake House near the medical center. With its old décor and sticky tables, their meal should pretty much guarantee diarrhea. TJ was nonstop talking, and I was barely listening. I had never had an MRI, and I had no idea what to expect.

We arrived at the medical center into a large waiting room that was full of people. *Are all of these people here for the same reason as me? Cancer? Hopefully, this will be fast, and maybe I can get a little retail therapy in before going home. This area does have far better shopping than my hometown. I want to make the best of this trip. Plus, we paid about $25 in tolls to get here.*

The nurse called me back and explained how the breast MRI was done. I would have part of the procedure done without dye, which would last twenty to thirty minutes and another twenty to thirty minutes with dye. They would need to start an IV for the dye. She explained that I would feel the coldness of the dye and told me not to worry. I was given a hospital gown to change into and special nonslip socks and a place to lock up all my clothes and purse. This was something that this nurse does every day, and she knew the routine well. After changing, she started the IV and looked like we were ready to go. She informed me that I would be lying on my stomach the entire time as there was no break in between the non-dye and the dye portion. I would lay flat with my breasts in a sort of boob holder, with my arms over my head. She reminded me not to move the entire time. Then she handed me earplugs because the machine could be very loud.

I put the earplugs in and lay down on the table. The techs would adjust me like I was a blob of Play-Doh that they could shape and mold. One of the techs gave me a button to push if I needed to get out for any reason. The machine guided me into the center of what seemed like a giant toilet paper tube. All I could hear was doors closing and the machine starting. As soon as I was in the machine, my right earplug fell out of my ear. "Oh shit, is this going to be a problem?" I never felt like I had an issue with small spaces. I had heard of people having panic attacks during an MRI, but that could not possibly happen to me. Small spaces didn't scare me; I was a regular at the tanning bed. If I could do that, then I know I could do this. I started to sweat and not just normal perspiration but sweating like I was about to pass out. I tried to close my eyes and just lay there to get it over with. The noise was overwhelming, and of course, I was down to one earplug. I finally could not take one more minute of it anymore. My chest was hurting, and I couldn't breathe. This was when I pushed the button. The tech came in, and I explained what was happening. It felt like hours that I was in the machine, but the tech let me know that I was in there for about seven minutes. Seven minutes! They were just getting started, and there was no way I could do this. The tech suggested that I come back another day and do this when I am calm. This was the breaking point for me. I could not comeback another day. My doctor needed this information now, and I needed to do this. This was when I started ugly crying. The tech asked if anyone was with me today. "Yes, my husband is in the waiting room." The tech left to get TJ as I cried. TJ came in the room, looking scared. What could have possibly gone wrong? The tech explained that I seemed to have a panic attack of sorts and needed something to take the edge off. The tech felt so bad for me that she said that she would get me done today, even if she worked through her lunch break. Before I knew it, she had called in a prescription for a muscle relaxer, and we could pick it up at the pharmacy around the corner from the medical center. The catch was that I would have to be present at the pharmacy to pick up the prescription. The tech told me to get dressed, but she would leave the IV in, and I was to knock on the back door instead of going through the waiting room again. Before I left for the prescription, she said that whatever I do, don't put anything in the IV. I was puzzled. What would I put in the IV?

"Oh, you know, heroin," she said rather matter-of-fact.

I assured her that me putting anything in that IV would not happen.

Getting the prescription was actually the easiest part of the day, and before I knew it, I was knocking on the back door of the medical center. The tech let us in and led us down a hallway. "Change back in the gown, take the medicine, and wait here. I will be back when I have an opening in the machine." TJ was sitting with me, watching *SportsCenter* on the television, as I was silently pondering what would happen next. I was so full of anxiety that even after thirty minutes, the prescription was not mellowing me out. I was having thoughts of what would happen if I had to get in this machine and I still could not do it. This was a procedure that I had to get done without exception. The tech returned, letting me know that apparently, the patient after me also had a freak-out moment and would be returning another day. That was great for me because it opened the time slot for me. Was I ready? I still was not feeling the relaxation that the prescription promised, so when TJ left to use the restroom and before the tech came to get me, I took another muscle relaxer. I planned to handle this MRI like a rock star. Little did I know that I was handling it like an '80s drug-fueled rock star who had no clue about what was going on.

The moment came, and down the hall I went to get this task done. TJ, channeling his former career as a high school football coach, gave me the "go get 'em" and "you can do this" pep talk. I was busy wondering why this muscle relaxer was not working.

In the machine I went . . . again. It was a very déjà vu moment. The earplugs went in, I was molded like Play-Doh, and into the large toilet paper roll I went. Even with the earplugs, the machine seemed really loud. The sounds started to run together in a pulsating rhythm. It reminded me of being at a dance club when I was in college, loud rhythms, bad lighting, and a little drunk. I stayed awake for the whole process. The dye running through the IV was cold, but it gave me hope that we were almost done. Finally, the machine stopped and the tech came in to announce that I could now move. I was stuck in the same position for so long that I was not sure that I could move at this point. TJ was waiting for me, and his face showed absolute pride. "You did it!" he exclaimed. My only response was "Yeah, I'm hungry now."

We got to the car, and I was busy telling TJ about how I didn't feel like the prescription worked. I expected to fall asleep but never did. Having never taken a muscle relaxer before, I was totally unaware that it was working, and since I took a second one before going in the MRI, it would continue working.

All I knew and could process at this point was that I needed food. I didn't remember my grand plans of shopping. TJ started with the question that every couple struggles with. Where do you want to go to eat? After a lot of back and forth, we agreed on sushi. The sushi restaurant was in a seedy part of town, but at this point, I just wanted food. We were seated and ordered, and things started to get a little blurry. TJ kept asking me if I was okay. I was okay, I think. Finally, I could not fight it anymore. My head went down on the table where it stayed while TJ finished his meal. I would like to say that I took a brief nap, but my face was on the table, and I was drooling. I think, at this point, the muscle relaxers had kicked in and were working. TJ helped me out to the car and got me home only to wake me up as we arrived at our house, making sure I was able to get up the stairs to bed.

Chapter 6

Who Wants to See Me Topless?

The remainder of the month of March, I showed my breast to more people than most strippers do in their entire career. The biggest difference is that they get tips for showing their breast and I am paying a co-pay. I had really tried to keep this situation out of the small-town rumor mill, but there was definitely no going around it. I had not been to work in a week because of all the appointments, and I was such a regular at the hospital that some people thought I worked there. There was the never-ending scans, MRIs, and meetings of the team that I would be trusting this journey to. It seemed as if every time I went to the cancer center, the patient outreach nurse was waiting for me with an appointment card for something else.

Other than that initial breast MRI, most of the scans were eventless. The usual needing of basic information and then take your top off. I was required to get a PET scan as my cancer was in my lymph nodes and the doctors wanted to make sure that it had not spread anywhere else. Once again, my small rural community did not have their own PET scan machine. It seemed like it was a machine that was not available at many of the hospitals near my area, so one hospital system had purchased a PET scan machine and put it in a refurbished travel camper. This camper was taken around to different communities for appointments. The patient outreach nurse gave me an appointment card that said it was at 7:30 p.m. an hour and a half away from my home. My first question was 7:30 p.m.? I had never heard of a doctor's office having evening hours like that before. The nurse reassured me that this was a legit situation and not to worry.

The day quickly arrived for this appointment, and I had my special prescription to help me just in case it was another giant toilet paper tube situation again. I followed all the procedures, such as no eating after 1:00 p.m. Once again, TJ agreed to make the trip with me just in case I needed the muscle relaxer. We were not quite sure where we were going, so we put the 911 address into our navigational system. The system took us to an almost-empty parking lot. There was a camper that was set up in the parking lot, and once I saw that, I immediately started laughing. In my hometown, the SPCA has an RV that comes around, called the Neuter Scooter. Is this lone camper in the parking lot like the Neuter Scooter? TJ and I got out of the car and looked around like we were lost. A lady came out of one of the buildings and asked if I were here for a PET scan and then reassured us that we were in the right place.

We went into the building but later found out that the prep work, such as an IV and drinking a really terrible chalk drink, were done there, but I would be moved to the camper which holds the scan machine. I looked around the waiting room, and for being after hours and a near-empty parking lot, the waiting room had a large number of people waiting around. I was taken back with another lady from the waiting room to a small closet. The lady with me went to another room. Shortly after sitting down, a young man entered the room and informed me that he was a nurse and would be starting my PET scan process by beginning an IV and getting me to ingest a special shake. This guy looked like one of my fourth graders! I felt like I was on an episode of *Doogie Howser, M.D.* I decided this was a great time to ask many questions: where he went to school, when did he graduate, did he always want to go into the medical field. The teacher in me came out, and it did not shake him one bit. Moments after the IV was in, the lady who came back with me from the waiting room was at the doorway with another nurse. She too had her IV in. The nurse asked if I minded if this lady joined me. Apparently, the PET scan area was backed up, and they needed a space to put people.

"The more, the merrier." I smiled and pointed to the chair next to me. The lady introduced herself as Ledeja. This was probably one of the most joyful moments of this experience. We sat and laughed like we were longtime girlfriends. Ledeja explained that she had stage 4 ovarian cancer. This was her second time around. She said that she thought she had beaten it the first time around, but that doesn't seem to be the case now. She talked about how her family is from the Bahamas and they had all kinds of suggestions on how to fight this cancer, none of which had any medical merit. After her first round with cancer, she did change the way she ate, cut out processed foods, ate organic, and drank green tea by the gallons. She was also a teacher and had worries about going back to work and being with her students. We both promised each other that we were going to fight hard because we are way too fabulous to die so young. Ledeja looked at me, smiled, and said, "Maybe we should smoke weed. I hear that it works for many cancer patients." We laughed and laughed at the vision of two straitlaced schoolteachers turning themselves into potheads.

I guess our laughing was echoing down the hallway because our young male nurse entered the room quickly, wanting to know if we were okay. Of course, we were okay. For two ladies facing life and death, we were doing pretty good. He brought with him the chalky shake that he had promised. Ledeja and I decided that we were going to chug it like we were at a college keg party. We laughed and then chugged it as fast as we could. It was horrible! We quickly realized that the PET scan shake is not meant to be taken in that manner. After finishing it off, we were escorted to the travel trailer outside. It was a quick walk, but a cold one. Inside were two recliners side by side, and we sat down and were given a warm blanket and the latest issue of *People* magazine. Ledeja was taken back first. We never saw each other after that. We did exchange phone numbers and text each other occasionally, but after a while, I had stop texting, and so had she. One day, I decided to text her and got the response that there was no one there with that name. My mind wandered, and I hoped that the reason no one was there with that name was because she got a new phone and lost her contacts. The worst did come to mind as well. She did have stage 4 cancer, and this was the second time. That was when the reality hit me that we all don't make it out of this club. This cancer club.

The PET scan was absolutely uneventful after that. It was not as cramped as the original MRI, and I was starting to feel like a professional when doing these scans. When I was free to leave, it was almost 10:00 p.m., and I was starving. Around the corner was a Jersey Mike's Subs shop. They were getting ready to close but waved us in. We went in to find many other people ordering subs at 10 p.m. as well. In the line, my mind was focused on the events of the day, the people I met, and some big scary thought about the PET scan. What I didn't notice at first was a woman staring at me. This woman was wearing what looked to be pajamas, with wild hair and an even wilder look in her eyes. She also reeked of alcohol.

"Hey, girl," she yelled across the Jersey Mike's line.

Is she talking to me?

"Hey, girl, I'm talking to you," she said again.

Oh shit, this woman is trying to start something with me. So I quickly looked at her and stood my ground. "Yes, do I know you?"

"No, girl, but I wanted to tell you that you are beautiful," she said with a bit of slurring.

I could not hold back a giggle and thanked her. I have always had a strong faith and belief in a higher power that will interact in your life at moments when you need it the most. I was surprised that God would send that message through a drunk woman at a Jersey Mike's, but it was exactly what I needed to hear at this moment. It seemed at that point on, I changed my perspective on this situation. The calmness of Ledeja and the not-so-calmness of this drunk woman made me realize that I have to handle this cancer with the finesse of both women. I need to take care of myself and push forward no matter the results I receive and have the flair to say what is on my mind and live my life. This is the time to tell people that you love them, forgive the people who have hurt you, and make the best of every day. Even though it is so cliché, it is true that tomorrow is not promised to anyone. TJ worked with a football coach years prior who would always say, "None of us are getting out of this alive." Truer words have not been spoken. He was right. We all face death at some point. I just wanted to make sure it was later and not sooner. There were so many things I needed to do, say, and see.

The next step in this process was finding out the path I would be taking to battle this cancer. I was finally going to meet the oncologist who would be working with me. It was a day of double appointments. I would first meet with the oncologist and then meet with the nurse practitioner to review the treatment schedule. TJ went with me to both appointments. The first was meeting Dr. Laura, my oncologist. I had already met the other oncologist, but he was retiring within days, so I was excited to meet the person whom I was going to be spending a lot of time with. She entered the room with a smile and reviewed the information from my file. She talked about a plan of chemotherapy first, surgery, and then radiation. The best-case scenario was for me to complete this in six months to a year. We also talked about how she was a chemistry teacher for a short period of time before going to medical school at the high school that my husband was once assistant principal. She was slightly older than us and was still in college when we were high school students and left before we started working for the schools. She was very optimistic with my treatment plan and felt that with my age and strength, I would do just fine in it. She did caution me with regard to my work. My first few chemotherapies were going to be tough, and the flu was going around at a record pace. She was concerned that working in an elementary school, I would be putting myself in harm's way. Her recommendation was to take time off from work so I could rest and recuperate.

"When should I start staying home? After the first chemo?"

"No, as soon as possible. You do not want to get sick prior to your treatment and cause a delay."

My cancer was aggressive, and I knew that I needed to get started as soon as possible. This was my first time with the Family Medical Leave Act paperwork, but throughout this journey, I found to be an expert in the process. My days were still going to filled with more appointments each day. I still had to meet with the surgeon who would put in my port, the breast surgeon who would remove my breasts, and the plastic surgeon who will rebuild my breasts.

I met with the nurse practitioner who was an absolute professional with reviewing the treatment medicines. I always get nervous when I am taken into little conference rooms at a hospital, and this moment was no different. In the future, I would always take note of when I see people go into the little room off the waiting room at the cancer center. It always gives me a bad feeling. I know what is happening there. It is a time of finding out the treatment plan and facing the scary and unknown. The NP named Jennifer was already with a neat binder with tabs and highlighted sections. Normally, the teacher in me would be excited to see this because for most educators, office supplies are exciting. I just could not bear to see what was inside this binder. She went over each page, discussing each type of chemotherapy medication, the side effects, and what to do when you have side effects. My first four treatments would be given with two different medications and fourteen days apart. The first medicine was named Doxorubicin, but I later learned its nickname, "the red devil." It was a bright-red fluid that the nurse would manually pump. It came with all kinds of great side effects, such as vomiting, diarrhea, mouth sores, and the big one, hair loss. This medicine was a devil, and I was going to get four chances to fight it. Along with this, I would take four cycles of Cyclophosphamide. This medicine was not nicknamed anything ominous, but it still was going to pack a punch.

After the first four cycles, I would go to every week with a combinations of Taxol, Herceptin, and Perjeta. The original plan was twelve cycles of these three medications. What I found out later was that I needed more than what was initially planned. Sitting and listening to the plan was a bit overwhelming. In my mind, I had not completely come to terms with my diagnosis. Hearing this was just too much for me, and I started to feel weak. The room was hot, and I was feeling like I could pass out at any moment. I think that the practitioner, Jennifer, noticed something was not right with me. I started using the binder she gave me to fan myself, so everything she was saying was basically going into one ear and out the other. Jennifer went to get me a water, and I immediately put my head down on the table. TJ was quick to ask if I was okay. My response was the same every time I get that question, "Just give me a minute. I will be okay."

I barely made it through that appointment. Before I made it out the door, the patient outreach worker was waiting for me with an appointment card for me to meet with a general surgeon. I was going to need a port before I start the chemo, and I should get it done in the next couple of days. This was so much I needed to process. I didn't even know what a port was and how it was used. My mother didn't have one when she went through chemotherapy.

The next day, I was sitting in the exam room, waiting for the general surgeon to meet with me. I went by myself because if TJ went with me to every appointment, he would never make it to work. This was just supposed to be a consultation, so it should be brief. The surgeon came in. He was an older gentleman with kind eyes, and I could tell that he enjoyed his job as a surgeon. He was quick to tell me all the benefits of a port and how he would put it in and even brought out a model of what a port looks and feels like under the skin. The problem was that once again, I was not listening. Actually, I was listening in the beginning, and just like the previous day, I was feeling faint. The room was hot, and it sounded like someone had their hands over my ears as everything was muffled. I don't think he noticed that I wasn't right because he finished what he was talking about and said something about the nurse coming back with my appointment information. The moment the surgeon and his nurse left the room, I lay down on the examination table. By the time the room stopped spinning, the nurse was back with a packet of information.

"You are in luck, Mrs. Johnson. The surgeon has a cancellation this Friday. You will need to go over to the hospital and register for your surgery as soon as possible. I would recommend that you do it as soon as you leave here," the nurse said.

Surgery in two days! This was the moment that I wish I had paid better attention during the appointment, but at least in my informational packet, there were brochures about what to expect.

Chapter 7

Easy Access

My days were all blending together. It seemed like my car was on autopilot and just automatically drove to the hospital campus each day. TJ went with me to drive me home. The packet of paperwork had me list the name of the person who was bringing me home before I was allowed to get the surgery. I was an early appointment, so I know that the surgeon wasn't running late. The nurse took me back quickly and said that TJ could come with me. This was becoming a routine of taking off my clothes and putting on the hospital gown and the nonslip socks that never seem to fit my big feet. The IV was started, and I waited for the party to begin. The surgeon stopped by to say good morning and go over what he planned to do. It seemed like he was reminding himself of what he needed to do. Before I knew it, the anesthesiologist was back and ready to push the good stuff into my IV. The nurses unlocked the wheels of the bed and started to roll me out the door and down the well-lit hallway to the surgery room. I remember the ceiling lights and the sound of the wheels on the floor, but I don't remember making it to the surgical room. Everything went dark.

When I woke up, I was back in the same room that I was in prior to the surgery, and TJ was sitting there, playing Candy Crush on his iPad. I was groggy and sore, with a big lump of bandages on my right side directly over my breast. The discharge nurse came in with a list of instructions. The big one was not to get the surgical area wet for two weeks. That instruction brought me out of my grogginess. How will I wash my hair? How will I wash my personal parts? I don't want to be funky! The nurse suggested sitting in a bathtub but waiting on the hair unless I have a washbasin with a chair like at a hair salon. She stressed that the surgical area cannot get wet under any circumstance as it could cause an infection which could be very serious.

TJ helped me get dressed, and the nurse returned with a wheelchair, ready to drop me off to the parking lot. TJ went ahead to bring the car around. The surgical nurse was young and very positive. She kept talking about what a good job I did and how once I start my chemo, I would really appreciate this port. Later on, I realized that she was right. The port was the way to go and made it possible for easy access to complete chemo and not burn out my veins. When the port was removed, two years later, I really missed it and found that my veins didn't want to behave when I had blood work or potassium infusions.

TJ was waiting in front of the hospital with the passenger door open and ready for me. I got in the car, and the exhaustion went over me like a wave. The ride home was short, but it felt like I had run a marathon and was in last place. My parents live in an apartment connected to our house and were waiting outside in the driveway when we pulled up. I had no time to talk. My goal was to put myself in my bed and sleep this nightmare away.

When I woke up, the bandages were still there, and the pain medicine was wearing off. The one thing that I always worried about was the dangers of opioid abuse. Having so many surgeries, I was always given prescriptions for pain medicine. I had watched enough episodes of *Intervention* to know that opioid abuse is real, and here I was with a lot of this medication in my possession. One thing that I learned about myself was that I didn't like the feeling of the pain medicine and would never finish a prescription. It gave me a feeling of being out of control, and my micromanaging self cannot stand to be out of control.

When I finally looked beneath the bandages, it was not too bad. There was bruising and some stitching, but the part that my eyes were automatically drawn to was the quarter-size lump directly below the stitching. I felt like the bionic woman. Well, maybe the bionic woman after losing a battle. The first couple of nights, it was difficult sleeping. I was not adjusted to the feeling of this extra equipment. The part that was most difficult for me was the bathing issue. This was going to be very challenging to not get this port wet for two weeks. I will admit that I am most definitely a shower person and do not have the patience to take a "luxurious bath." Another issue would be the washing of hair. I could go two days or so without washing my hair, but two weeks would be a definite stretch. I started to feel itchy just thinking about this. I did everything I could to not get the port wet. I only filled the bathtub with about two to three inches of water, covered the port area with cling wrap, and was extremely cautious. Still, getting out of the tub, I did not feel clean. After several days, I broke down and called the young woman who cuts and colors my hair. I explained the situation to her, and she fit me in between appointments to get my hair washed and blown out. I did this once a week for the time that I was unable to take a shower. My last couple of weeks of having hair, and I must admit, it looked damn good.

I had one more major appointment that had to be taken care of before starting the chemotherapy, and that was an echocardiogram. It was needed to make sure that my heart could withstand the stress and strain of chemotherapy. Once again, this was a procedure that was completely foreign to me. I had always been relatively healthy before this diagnosis. The thought of getting an echocardiogram seemed to be a procedure that was reserved for old people, not someone my age, but here I was waiting to do this. I didn't understand the significance of this appointment until months later, but it had a huge impact on me and defined the relationships that I made through this journey.

The echo tech was a woman around my age. She was very personable and engaged me into conversation quickly. Living in a small community, if you do not directly know someone, you figure out people you both know to draw a connection. We figured out our connection quickly as she went to the prom with one of my husband's high school friends. We talked about our families, where our kids go to school, and what brought me to the hospital for this procedure. One thing that stood out in my mind through our entire conversation was that I told her that if she ever found any lumps or bumps around her breasts or in her armpits, to get it checked out. I enjoyed talking with her and told her that I would see her in around six months for my next echo. Little did I know that I would see her sooner than later. Months into my chemo treatment, I was sitting in the cancer center waiting room, awaiting my time for my treatment, when the door to the little room, the room that I learned my cancer plan, opened, and out walked the echo tech. She was with her husband and an older woman, who I thought was possibly her mother. All three looked upset and understandably so because I know the purpose of that little room. At the time, I assumed that maybe her mother or her husband was sick. I found out later, after running into her in the community, that shortly after my echo, she found a lump in her breast. It hurt my heart that another young woman was initiated into this terrible cancer club.

I had already had two friends in the cancer club: my friend Laura, whom I would see at the YMCA and at events at the local Elks Lodge, and then my friend Melissa, who owned a local beauty salon. These were active young women who practiced healthy habits. How could this happen? Melissa had a double heartache with cancer as the day she was diagnosed, so was her mother. Now I was facing a new young woman who would be embarking on this wild journey. Little did I know that throughout my journey, I would be welcoming three more of my friends to the club. It always hurt my heart to hear the news, but in some odd way, their journey helped me get through the rough days, and maybe I did the same for them. We would all communicate through text messages or Facebook Messenger to get information. Melissa and Laura were my go-to for a lot of information because they were ahead of me with their diagnosis. Even though everyone has a different journey, there are many similarities, and that was enough to give me some peace of mind when starting a new treatment or having a procedure completed.

I met so many survivors at the cancer center. Many of the volunteers were survivors of cancer, and it was important for them to give back and be a support team to people entering their journey. All the health-care workers who had dedicated their life to helping cancer patients were always there with a smile or encouraging words. Also, going through treatment, I met so many people in the same situation as me. We talked, laughed, and sometimes cried. I was never alone through this whole process, even when there were times when I thought that I wanted to be alone. I had the support of my family and friends, but now I had this whole new group of people cheering me on to the finish line. The trick for now is to make it to the finish line.

Chapter 8

The Devil Is Real and Red

While I waited for my port to heal enough to access, I was sequestered to my home. The purpose was to avoid the flu so that I could get my treatment started. Time was of the essence since my cancer showed to be active and ready to spread around my body. I felt good physically. The lump was still there, and multiple times each day, I would touch it. I felt like I was playing hooky from school since I was home and felt fine. The big picture of the situation was that I needed to avoid getting sick so that I could move forward. Meanwhile, I caught up on every episode of every town of *The Real Housewives*. I still had not made it official knowledge what was happening. Since my job had me at a different school each day, it was easy to fall off the radar of some of my colleagues, but eventually, it would be public knowledge that I would be out on medical leave. TJ was asking when I was going to make it official, and in this time of social media, one would make it Facebook official. I was not at the point in my illness that I was able to say out loud "I have breast cancer" without crying. The moment finally presented itself. I was scrolling Facebook, and the hospital was advertising my two doctors. Dr. Laura and my future radiologist, Dr. Jefferson, were presenting a forum on making the community aware of the local cancer center. This was my moment. I shared the status and wrote, "My doctors who are working with me as I start my breast cancer journey." There . . . it was officially out there. My phone buzzed all night with comments and text messages. I cried a lot that night, but I knew that there was a community of support, and I knew that one thing I had to do was accept help.

The day finally came. The port area was healed, and I was scheduled for the first chemotherapy. I was given a prescription of a topical numbing ointment that would go over the port. I was to put it on the port area about a half hour before my appointment and cover it with plastic wrap to warm up the area and activate the ointment. It was all worked out that I would go to chemo with my mother and TJ would come by at lunchtime to bring lunch. The cancer center only allowed one person at a time, but TJ was able to sneak in, bringing lunch, and check on me. It gave my mom time to go the restroom and stretch her legs. I didn't know what to pack, and I have always had a habit of over packing. I knew that I would be there the entire day, but what would I need? I definitely over packed and learned my lesson for the next thirty-nine treatments. I had a huge LLBean boat bag filled with a blanket, pillow, book, candy, and computer. I don't think I used anything in the bag because the cancer center thought of everything.

I was taken back to the infusion lounge and placed in the cubicle directly in front of the nurse's station. The newbies were always placed there to monitor any possible reactions. My nurse was Stephanie, and she was exactly the type of person I needed to be around at this moment. She was a feisty redhead who just had a fun aura. I knew her children as they used to babysit Madison and Morgan when they were little but didn't really know her until now. On this first day, I didn't understand how important Stephanie and the rest of the nurses in the infusion lounge would be to me. I learned very quickly that these people were going to be important, just like my own family.

Stephanie was cheerful and explained everything that she was going to do and brought out a tray of all the equipment that she would use to access my port. She promised that this would be a short time of being uncomfortable to access the port and then everything would be great. She was right. It was a little pinch and a little pressure on the spot, and I was all hooked up. There was a reason this was going to be an all-day process since chemo was a slow infusion, plus the number of bags I had to go through each time. The first bag was a saline solution to flush the port and prepare for the chemo. This was going to be the first half hour. This saline flush was actually a cruel trick. It was cold, and I had no discomfort. In my mind, I kept thinking if this was how it would be, then it would be pretty easy. Then things changed. Stephanie came back and said in her cheery voice that my first bag of chemo had arrived from the hospital pharmacy and she was going to "suit up" and get it started. When she meant "suit up," it meant putting on what looked like a hazmat suit. She also brought with her another nurse from the department. The purpose of the extra nurse was to read the prescription information from the infusion bag and confirm that in fact, I was receiving the correct chemotherapy. Many questions flooded my mind. *Why don't I get a special suit? If the nurses have to wear this, is it safe to put in my veins?*

I tried to put everything out of my mind. It was hard to not listen to the clicking of the infusion machine or the random beeping. My mom was sitting with me, and she was doing her best to be upbeat. Her eyes told it all. She was worried and also reflecting on her own cancer experience. She said several times how things were so different when she went through the process. I had to clear my mind, so what better way than to watch television. Each cubicle had a recliner, a chair for a guest, and a television. I flipped through the channels, and there were news, sports, and Disney channels. I finally found the mindless television that was going to help me try to forget the chemical that was steadily pumping into my port. My chemo savior was none other than *Dog the Bounty Hunter*. It took my mind off everything that was going on. For forty chemo sessions, Dog and I had a standing date. I also became obsessed with the shows *Hoarders* and *My 600-lb Life*. Mindless television was the way I was going to take the focus off the constant push of chemicals into my veins. Once again, God sent me a savior with over bleached hair, bad jewelry, and feathers in his hair.

The moment that the red devil was to be administered, it did not come in a bag like the other chemo. This time, it came in a large syringe. It was definitely red. Stephanie explained that it had to be manually pumped and it was pumped slowly to watch for side effects. One thing that the nurses were watching for was if I were to get chills. Not just chills like I am a little cold. This was chills likes teeth chattering and uncontrollable shivering. The devil started, and I was starting to get chills. Stephanie kept bringing me warmed blankets, and I was wrapped up like a mummy, but I was not to the extent that they did not feel that I could continue.

I had made it through the first infusion and just felt tired. My mind swirled with wonder of what would I feel like in an hour, twelve hours, or twenty-four hours. Before I could leave, there was one more thing that needed to be done. Stephanie said that I was to get a Neulasta shot. This was supposed to help keep my platelets at a healthy level and allow me to be strong enough during the effects of the devil. I had seen commercials for Neulasta. Everyone in the commercial looked happy. They were fishing, doing yoga, and going to flea markets. How bad could this be since everyone in the commercial seemed like it was the miracle that would get you through chemotherapy?

Stephanie brought all the materials and started to set everything up. She explained that she would stick it to a fatty area and start the timer and a needle would inject. After about twelve hours, the medication in the on-body container would automatically inject the medication. I would have to wait several hours after the dispensing of the medication, and then I was to remove the on-body container. This entailed me having to pull the needle out. I was not sure if this was something that I could handle.

The moment arrived, and Stephanie put it on the fatty section on the back of my arm. She stuck it firmly to my arm and then turned a dial. It immediately started clicking. It reminded me of an old-fashioned kitchen timer. *Tick, tick, tick, tick,* and then I felt the needle quickly inject in my arm. I think I may have screamed out a little. It was a machine that beeped and had lights that would blink, so there was no way of being inconspicuous with this thing. Stephanie explained all the procedures of how to take care of it. I was not ready, but I really didn't have a choice at this point.

I sat in a chair all day, talking to Mom and watching television, but I was exhausted. The moment I arrived home, I was ready to go to bed. TJ's cousin brought dinner to the house, and I felt like a terrible hostess because I could barely stay awake to talk. The worst was sitting there waiting to see what kind of symptoms I would experience. Two things happened from that first chemo. The first was that my urine was neon orange, and the second thing was that all food and drink tasted like metal. Everything tasted like old nickels, not that I chew on old nickels as a hobby.

The first few days were uneventful, and I got the false sense of security that this would not be so bad. The Neulasta on-body injector did what it was supposed to do. It started to beep, and then I could hear the medication release. I had to wait a couple of hours before I could remove the on-body equipment, and that was definitely a concern. I would be the first to admit that I can be a bit of a wimp, and the idea of pulling that needle out had me scared and nervous. This was something that I would have to do a total of four times, so I had better get adjusted to it. The moment arrived, and I had to sit down so that I could do this without fainting. It was not as bad as I expected, but I learned that the Neulasta commercials are basically a big lie. I did not feel like doing yoga or visiting a flea market as the actors were shown in the commercial. The reality of the situation was that I could not get out of bed. I didn't want to eat, and it was challenging just having the energy to walk down the stairs. The time that I started to feel better was about two days before my next treatment.

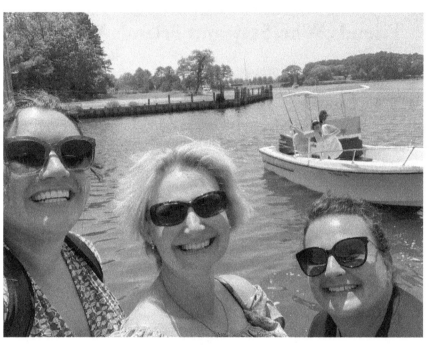

(A day with friends; Left to Right Christy Ann, Becky, Karrie)

Chapter 9

Friends Who Stay and Friends Who Go

My friend Christy Anne said to me once, when someone is diagnosed with an illness or there is a death in the family, there seems to be this morbid fascination from some people. It is like when someone in your family dies, and for about a week, you are overrun with cakes and casseroles, but after that week, those same people have moved on to the next traumatic event. Finding out you are ill is really an eye-opening experience of who truly cares for you and who just really enjoys the drama. I also found some people who seemed jealous of the fact that I was receiving attention. I can honestly say that people whom I have always put first in my life suddenly couldn't be bothered with me and people whom I may not have known as well turned out to be the most loving and caring individuals in my life.

An example is my friend Jaime, whom I have known for over a decade. Our children are the same age, except she has two boys and I have two girls. We met in the Mommy and Me swim classes at the local YMCA with our oldest children. Jaime works in the same school division as me and had a position similar to me where she travels to different schools. Jaime and I are friends. When I see her out, we speak, but that was it. The day after I made my diagnosis "Facebook official," she had organized a meal train for my family. For about four to five months, she had organized someone bringing my family dinner each evening. When someone was unable to complete the obligation, Jaime stepped in and took over their night. I was so touched by this gesture that in everything that was happening to me, I could never forget all she did for me. How do you "pay back" the gesture? I honestly don't think I can ever pay her back for everything she did for my family, as well as the people who participated in making sure my family was fed every evening. There were days when I could not even get out of bed, and if I did not have this support, I would also have the worry of what my family was eating. Now don't get me wrong, TJ is a great husband, cook, and father, but we have always been a team, and when one team member is down, the game gets harder to play.

The thing that also struck me was the list of people who had signed up. They were doing this from their heart and their concern for me and my family. Another thing that struck me was the people who were missing. People whom I had spent lots of time with, gone on vacations with, and shared important events with were nowhere to be found. Those were the same people that I barely heard from. It hurt me at first and for quite a while. TJ would tell me that not everyone has the same heart. I would get so mad and call them garbage humans. How could they watch me and my family go through this, and the most I would get from them is the prayers emoji on Facebook when TJ would update my condition? I felt forgotten, but TJ was very quick to remind me of the wonderful people who were there for us for the long haul, not the novelty of the event and waiting for the next tragedy to happen to someone else.

This group of wonderful people helped get my family over the hump. That was something that I can say was a positive thing about having cancer. I learned who my real friends are and who are just fair-weather friends. It was hard. There were things I was not invited to because who the hell wants to party with a chemo patient? Another thing was going out, and every time I would run into someone, they wanted to talk cancer. In my head, I was screaming, "There is more to me than cancer," but then I quickly realized that at this moment, I was all about cancer.

Another thing that I learned quickly was to filter out the negative people. For example, when someone comes to you and says, "Yeah, my mother had breast cancer, and she died from it really fast." These are the people one must stay away from. I'm in the fight of my life, and I don't want to hear the story of your family member who lost that battle. The people I started to surround myself with are the warriors, the people who kick-ass and take names. Some of these people I had no clue went through this battle. They just kept it to themselves and kept on stepping.

Like I said earlier, there are people in your life who are just your tribe. They care for you no matter what. It is important to cherish those people. Two of my friends from high school and on, Krysten and Traci, came and sat with me during one of my treatments. They took off work to sit and watch some machine pump chemicals into me. I know that it was pretty alluring to sit for hours to watch *Dog the Bounty Hunter*, but I truly believe that being with me during treatment was more important than Dog's bizarre story line.

This entire experience made me look at people differently. A person whom I knew for twenty years and who worked with my husband never asked how I was doing until she had to face me one day. It is hard to avoid the topic when I looked like an extra from the Walking Dead and was completely bald. This was a person whom I knew for so long and went on vacations with her family and who threw me a wedding shower when I married TJ, and all I could get was "How are you?" Part of me wanted to guilt her and say something like "Hope I can make it to next week" or "What do you mean, do I look sick or something?" When it would upset me, TJ would remind me that people like her are garbage. Yes, that is harsh, but some people are so self-absorbed that they cannot even fathom showing compassion and empathy to someone else. People like this taught me an important lesson. The lesson was to never be like them. I don't care how many Sundays you sit in a church pew and say amen; when you cannot care to reach out to someone going through the biggest fight of their life, you are garbage.

An important part of this journey, is coming out of it a better person. Before this, I could probably fall into the self-absorbed category.

I was all about just my family and close friends. I suddenly valued every conversation with every person that I met on this journey. My own children would get mad because I could not make it through basic grocery shopping in the local Walmart in less than one to two hours. Why? It was because I would run into people and end up in big conversations. On days that I was really sick, TJ would do the grocery shopping, and he had the same issue.

The best part is learning about the people who truly care for you, whether it is the friend who creates a meal train, the people who bring meals, the neighbor who would make flower arrangements from her flower garden each week and just put them in the house while I was resting, or the people who just want to sit and talk. Embrace those people because they are going to help you make it through this. Once I reach the side of recovery, my goal is to be just as compassionate, caring, and giving as these people.

Chapter 10

Jenny from the Block and Teddy

I met a lot of doctors, physician assistants, nurses, techs, and more in my cancer travels. The people who will be the biggest part of one's life will always be those who "broke the news to you," the oncologist, and the radiologist. Plus, I had a special bond with the nurses in the infusion lounge because, of course, they spent a lot of time with me.

There were two more people who played a big role in this cancer show, and it was the breast surgeon and the plastic surgeon. It had already been decided that the left breast needed to be removed because of the cancer. My right breast apparently knew how to behave, but I decided to have it removed as well. I had several fears about the breast removal. One reason was very logical, and one was purely superficial. The logical reason was the fear of going through this whole process of removing the left breast, and fast forward through the years, I have to go through it again with cancer in the right breast. The purely superficial reason was if I get one breast removed, even with an implant in the left, they would not look right. Not that I am actively flashing them around for all to see, but I look in the mirror, and my husband would see them. Do I want one perky, sitting high, perfectly shaped breast and one droopy, "breastfed two children" breast that looks like a tube sock with a marble at the end? No! I want them both to look like twenty-year-old breasts on an old lady. I want to look good in my shirts and have a little cleavage.

I had never considered plastic surgery before this journey. Yes, I had seen commercials of plastic surgeons advertising the "mommy makeover," which gives you back your "hot body" after having children. TJ would always joke that if I had one more baby and it was a son, he would spring for the mommy makeover. I would always joke back that this baby machine is closed and we only know the recipe for making girls, so get over it. I see women on television who get fillers all over, and I watch the show *Botched* about people who get really bad plastic surgeries, women and men who go to foreign countries to get cheaper rates or just go to surgeons who do not have their patients' best interest at heart.

All of a sudden, I was immerged in a world that I knew nothing about. First, I had to find a surgeon that could remove the breasts in manner that reconstruction can be put together with a minimum of difficulty. There are surgeons everywhere, but do they know how to properly demo a woman's breast? Dr. Laura had suggestions, and we had built a relationship, so I definitely trusted her opinion. One of her suggestions was a woman surgeon, Dr. Jenny. The appointment was made, and the plan was to be made on my mastectomy.

Dr. Jenny is a breast surgeon. She does not work on any other parts. Breasts are her specialty. I took my mom with me to meet her. It was difficult to wrap my mind around the impeding surgery and all of the what-ifs of the situation. After registering at the front desk, a nurse greeted me and said that Dr. Jenny would be doing an ultrasound and then meeting with me to review the plan. I felt even better that my mom was allowed to go to the ultrasound room as well. Mom and I sat in the ultrasound room alone, me in my paper vest (opened to the front as always) and Mom looking like a nervous wreck but trying to hold it together for me.

The door flung open really fast, and all of a sudden, I heard, "Hey, cutie patootie." I have never been addressed by a doctor like that and was taken a little off guard. She was my age and seemed like she was going one hundred miles per hour all the time. She was upbeat and positive. That was what I needed at that moment. I needed someone to take the dark cloud over my head and brighten my day. She gave me hope at a time I really needed it. On the flip side, she was very thorough and upfront about what was happening and what the future was going to look like. She did the ultrasound and gave lively commentary throughout the process. She noted how I definitely have a breast that was not behaving. Dr. Jenny spent time looking carefully at the breast at all different angles and taking pictures. Even though she had this very casual demeanor, I instantly felt comfortable and trusted her knowledge.

"All righty, you definitely have a bad boob, but it is nothing we cannot handle. Go ahead and get dressed and we will meet in my office to go over the plan."

I dressed quickly because I was curious of the next steps with surgery. *Will I lose my breast? Will it look like a Franken-boob?* The thoughts going through my head were big and scary. I was trying to pull it together to not worry my mom, and she was trying to look positive for my sake.

I got myself together, and my mom and I went directly to Dr. Jenny's office. She had a binder put together with my pathology reports and surgery information. Dr. Jenny was holding the binder as if she were ready to do a presentation.

She started with "You are ER (estrogen receptors) positive but barely. You are PR (progesterone receptors) negative and Her2 positive (the cancer tested positive for the human epidermal growth factor receptor 2 protein). You will be starting your chemotherapy. After your last THP (docetaxel, trastuzumab, and pertuzumab) chemo, we will wait one month and have surgery. For the surgery, I will remove both breasts, and during the surgery, the plastic surgeon will come in and put in tissue expanders. You will be meeting the plastic surgeon that I work with next week. Your treatment plan will continue after the surgery with radiation therapy. This will be about fifteen-minute sessions for five days a week for six weeks. Then you will be on a hormonal therapy, preferably Tamoxifen for five to ten years. Hormonal therapy will kick you into menopause with all kinds of fun things like hot flashes and vaginal changes."

She then talked cancer and sex. That was a bit awkward with my mother sitting there. Yes, I am married and have two children, so it is obvious that I have sex, but I wasn't planning that discussion in front of my mother. Dr. Jenny did not sense my awkwardness. She kept on talking about all these medications and treatments and how they can cause extreme vaginal dryness. She recommended the best brand of lubricants that can help. I followed her advice like it was the Gospel, but chemotherapy and sex do not go together. Regardless of all the brands of lubricants, sex was painful. She also suggested that all sexual contact should have use of a condom. Here I am in my forties, in almost a two-decade relationship, having a condom talk with a doctor. Her concern was the strong medications in the chemo prescriptions causing complications for my husband such as burns. The look on my mother's face was basically like she just wanted the floor to open up and swallow her up. Not only does she have to listen to her daughter going through a very intense cancer treatment but also listen to a sex talk.

Finally, it was over, with the next follow-up appointment scheduled. Surgery would be planned for late August or September. Mom and I just sat in the car, overwhelmed with information and another binder filled with lots of handouts, diagrams, and charts. I still had not grasp the fact that I have cancer, so understanding all this information was not sinking in. I figured that if I just look like I understand, then everyone will stop talking, and all of this will go away.

I knew the moment that I met Dr. Jenny that she was the surgeon for me. Everyone had recommendations, and I had countless people tell me to get a second opinion. I respect that some people want multiple opinions, but all the doctors I have met with have given me no reason to doubt them. They all backed up their diagnosis with pathology reports. Plus, time was not on my side. I knew the aggressiveness of the cancer I was dealing with. The time it takes to doctor shop may cause me bigger problems than I originally started with. Dr. Jenny proved to me that she was the right surgeon for me. Plus, she was a big personality, which I liked because sometimes I could be a big personality too. Over my time as her patient, she earned the nickname "Jenny from the block." One of her other patients and a friend of mine Stephanie found out that Dr. Jenny had attended a Flo Rida concert and ended up dancing with him onstage. She was also known at the surgical center for playing hip-hop music during surgeries. Yes, I wanted the rock star surgeon, and her performance in the operating room matched her personality.

The next person on the never-ending list of medical professionals was the plastic surgeon, Dr. Teddy. He was the surgeon that Dr. Jenny tag teams with on the reconstruction of breasts for cancer patients. This was an appointment that TJ was overly excited to attend. I think that he thought he was going to see pictures of breasts or maybe get to hold implants. When people think of plastic surgeons, many think Hollywood and that zest to attain the look of perfection. Even I thought that the waiting room would be full of beautiful people and trophy brides getting ready for bikini season. I was far from correct. The waiting room had people who were just like me, needing some sort of reconstruction, women who were going through treatments. Maybe the strippers and trophy brides were scheduled for another day because they certainly were not there on my appointment dates. One thing that stood out to me about this office was how it was run like a well-oiled machine. Everything ran on time, and I barely had time to fill out the new patient paperwork before the nurse was calling me and TJ back. Since this was a new experience, I just wanted to take everything in. The nurse went through the usual routine of undress from the waist up, with the paper vest open to the front. I had done this so much that I started before she even exited the room.

Dr. Teddy entered the room, introduced himself, and quickly went straight to work, opening the paper vest and moving my breasts around. TJ was quiet and watching as the doctor manipulated my breasts, feeling the lumps that originally caused this, giving directions and measurements to the nurse, even to the point of folding my breasts like he was closing an envelope. This was not the sexy side of plastic surgery. This was more like someone putting Humpty Dumpty back together again.

It felt surreal until the moment that Dr. Teddy said, "What are we doing about your nipples? Do you want me to reconstruct them?"

Honestly, that was not something that had been a focus point for me. Yes, I knew that I was going to lose my left nipple because it had been invaded by cancer, but I didn't even imagine what I would look like or how to remedy the situation and look normal. My mind was full of questions. How do you "make" nipples? Is it like a fondant flower on a cake? What does that look like? Another option was three-dimensional nipple tattoos. How will that look, and where do I find someone to do it and do it right?

I must have had a crazy look on my face and looked completely dazed because Dr. Teddy was quick to say, "We have time to think about what you want to do. Think about what you would like to do, and we will continue the conversation. As we get closer to the surgery date, we will work out the details of what to do. You will initially receive tissue expanders because the radiation will shrink the skin, and we will need to do some stretching before the actual implant can be put in. I promise you that you are going to be happy with the results."

"Can you make my breasts look better than now?"

"Yes, I can help you and will do everything to make you feel confident and happy."

I felt good leaving the appointment, but I could see the uneasiness on TJ's face. In the car, we drove for a while and finally broke the silence.

"What is the matter, TJ?"

"I like him, but it is difficult to see a man touching your breasts."

"Really, it is his job. He probably looks at breasts all day, and they all blend together." I laughed.

"Yeah, but you are my wife," TJ said.

"He is helping me."

"I get that and think that he is a great doctor, but this is a lot to take in," TJ said.

The drive home was full of discussion of what the next steps would be. Once again, I had met a doctor who was proving to be the ultimate professional, but sometimes the fear of the unknown could get in the way. TJ did not go back to those plastic surgery appointments. He did go to the surgeries and thinks highly of Dr. Teddy, but sometimes our fears of this process manifest in different ways. For TJ, it became real at the plastic surgeon's office. Even though TJ had seemed to accept the diagnosis early on, this appointment and this day was when I think it became real to him. This would begin a long relationship with Dr. Teddy in this crazy journey.

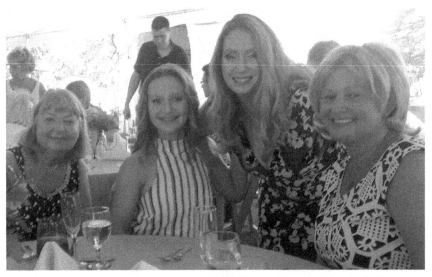

(Trying to be normal at my cousin's wedding Left to Right;
Pat (Becky's Mom), Madison, Noelle (Becky's cousin), and Becky

Chapter 11

Wigging Out

One of the side effects of the red devil is hair loss. The paperwork that I received that described the chemotherapy said "possible hair loss." After the first treatment, my long hair was still there, and I started to think that maybe I dodged having hair loss. Several days after the second treatment, it happened, and it happened fast. I ran my hands through my hair, and it came out in big clumps. I stood in my bedroom with two handfuls of long blonde hair. I had to decide. Do I just keep going through day after day, waking up with a pillow covered in hair and touching my head for clumps to fall out, or do I take care of it once and for all and shave my head?

I didn't even think about the hair loss. The cancer center tried to prepare me for that, but I was so delusional that I didn't even really ponder what I was going to do. In my "Welcome to the Cancer Center" bag, there was a catalog from the National Cancer Society filled with head coverings and wigs. I finally went back to that bag and unearthed that catalog. Originally, I thought that I would be a constant wig wearer. My friend Melissa, who was going through treatment, had a wig that looked so much like her hair that I was unsure that she had even lost her hair. She is a hairstylist and had the skills to make this work. Me, I can barely style my own hair, more or less transform a wig. I didn't even know proper wig etiquette.

If you are ever shopping for a wig, know that two types are available. The first type is an '80s news broadcaster/*Falcon Crest* TV show extra or hooker. The hooker wigs were actually more appealing and looked like they were more fun to wear. I had in my mind that I wanted many wigs and to change my look up on different days. I couldn't even make up my mind on a wig, so my mother stepped up to the plate and found a wig that looked very much like my own hair. When I looked in the mirror, I thought it looked like my normal self. Unfortunately, that was not so for others as people I had known forever didn't recognize me or were wondering who that woman was that TJ showed up with. It was me . . . in a wig. I looked like the extra from *Falcon Crest*.

The thing about the wig, for me, was that I felt like everyone could tell it was a wig. Was it on straight? Looking back on pictures of myself, I saw me . . . in a wig. It didn't look natural and didn't feel right to me. It was itchy and hot. I tried all sorts of advice to make it work, but I was not patient enough to make it work. I ended up embracing the bald life. My morning routine was so much shorter. I did learn that I had to up my makeup game because I didn't want to go around looking like a cancer patient. One of the must-have items was what I called my buggy cap. It was a soft cotton cap that hugged my head just right. I had many of these caps, but my two favorites were the navy blue one and the black one. I had bought many caps and hats, but nothing felt as nice as the buggy caps. I even had elastic headbands that went over the caps if I wanted to jazz up my look. I would wear a wig when going out to a restaurant or an event. I didn't want to draw attention to myself with a shiny bald head or even with the buggy caps.

Getting bald was certainly an adventure. TJ said that I needed to figure out what I wanted to do after several days of pulling out chunks of hair. Did I want to beat the punch and shave my head? When my mother went through cancer treatment, I encouraged her to shave her head. Melissa was the one who did that for my mother. She met us at her salon on a Sunday so my mom would have privacy. I remember it being a tearful moment. Now Melissa was going through her own cancer struggle. I could have reached out to my own ladies who do my hair, but part of me didn't want anyone to see me so vulnerable. Could

I do this myself? What about letting TJ shave my head? He had offered, but even though we have shared everything, I was not ready to put him through that. He had an idea. He called his cousin Amber. She had been in the hair and makeup business for years. She agreed to come over and shave my head.

I decided that this was going to happen at a time when the girls were at school and TJ was at work. My mom came over. It seemed like a déjà vu, except this time my head was getting shaved. Amber showed up with her bag of tools to make this happen. We did this in the kitchen with a drop cloth on the floor and a towel around my neck. She started slow, and I watched what was left on my head falling to the floor. I started to feel weak and faint. Amber stopped, and I went and lay down on the sofa with a fourth of my head bald. *Why am I feeling this way? It is only hair.* Losing my hair was the opening of the floodgates of emotion. My crown was being knocked off my head, and now it was time to fight. The reality hit me. It took longer than usual for Amber to shave my head. I had to go back and forth to the sofa to lie down. When I would go lie down, I would hear Amber and Mom whispering. They were worried about how I was handling this. Was the shaving of the head too soon? Was it finally sinking in my brain what was happening?

I made it through the head shaving, which seemed like an eternity. That first look in the mirror, I tried not to cry, but I did. *Who is this bald woman? Is she going to make it through this?* Amber and Mom were emotional too. Amber gave me a quick hug and told me that she was there for me. I was grateful for her help because I knew that I could not do that by myself and I could not have done it in public. I sat in the living room, thinking about what Madison, Morgan, and TJ will say when they see me. This was more than "I changed my hairstyle."

TJ had picked the girls up from school and had warned them on the car ride home what had happened. The moment they saw me, they had this look of shock. *Who is this woman?* I tried to act upbeat. I definitely did not want to cry in front of them. I joked about how I was rocking this look. The one thing that was important to me was that I did not want my children to feel my pain. I did not want them to see me cry or show any sign of weakness. I also did not want to embarrass them.

Being a teenager is hard enough, and now they have a cancer patient mom who has a shiny bald head. Madison was curious and had lots of questions. She wanted to feel my head and asked about when it would grow back and if it felt weird. Morgan, on the other hand, was shrinking back. There was fear, but she just didn't want to talk about it.

The hair on my head was not the only hair that I lost. When you lose your hair, you lose your hair everywhere! I lost the hair on my head, my eyebrows, my eyelashes, my pubic hair, and my leg and arm hair. The most traumatic was not the hair on my head even though I was so worried about that. It was the loss of my nose hair. One might laugh and say, "What is so traumatic about nose hair?" Let me tell you that your nose hair is important and serves important purposes. It is a defense system, it keeps harmful stuff out of your nose like dust and debris, and it maintains important moisture from the air that we breathe in. So yes, nose hair is important. Without nose hair, I had a runny nose that would not stop. I constantly had Kleenex with me because it just would not stop. There was nothing there to stop it. It was so bad that sometimes the mucus would just drip down my face because I couldn't even feel it happening. This will give you strange looks in social situations, and I advise always having a tissue in your hand, pocket, or bag. Of my hair loss situation, the only hair that did not grow back was my nose hair and my eyelashes.

My eyelashes grew back . . . somewhat. They grew back uneven and stubby. To this day, I am always using strip lashes or debating eyelash extensions. I was so weak at the time that I did not realize that my eyebrows and eyelashes were gone. One day, when I was feeling good, TJ had suggested going out. I was excited to get out of my pajamas, leave the house, and enjoy a spring day. I started to get ready with my usual routine, and that was when I realized the absence of the brows and lashes. It changed the whole look of my face. I looked ill, and it was hard looking in the mirror.

One day, on the way to my cousin's wedding in New Jersey with my mom and Madison, I was lamenting about how I look like a cancer patient. From the back seat, Madison chirped, "Well, do something about it."

Okay, but what can I do? I had no clue how to make myself look less cancer patient-ish. Madison's suggestion was to stop by the Ulta makeup supply store on our way to New Jersey. I really did not want to look ill for the wedding. I didn't want my family looking at me and worrying. This was an exciting event, and I didn't want to be the wet blanket. My northern family knew I was sick, but I was always upbeat on social media and never posted pictures of myself. I was not sure what my mom was telling them, so goodness knows what they were expecting. We stopped at an Ulta, and one of the salespeople directed me to their "eye salon" where they do waxing (not needed) and lashes. She put on individual lashes and taught me how to draw on my own eyebrows. I felt like a diva when I left. Finally, I looked somewhat back to normal. The trick was that I needed to keep these lashes on for the wedding the next day. The lady promised that these lashes were good for about four weeks. I must have done something wrong because the next morning (even though I slept on my back the entire night), the lashes were all wonky, half on, half off. *What am I going to do?* Madison rushed in for the save again by suggesting going to an Ulta here in New Jersey.

Now let me be clear, I am not trying to stereotype anyone, but there is a clear difference in the cosmetologist at a Maryland Ulta and a New Jersey Ulta. There seems to be a little more emphasis on the glamorous in the New Jersey stores, or at least the one I visited. The lady assisting me was dressed like she was ready for some sort of night club activity, lots of hair and lots of makeup. I explained my situation, and she helped to get the remaining lashes off and went to work doing my makeup for the wedding. I did have to remind her that I was not her age, so the makeup should be for a woman in her forties. When we got to the lashes, she showed me how easy it was to apply and remove strip lashes and immediately showed how she was wearing two pairs of lashes because she liked the volume.

Nervously, I reminded her of my age. I told her that I just wanted to look normal. Apparently, normal looks like a retired Vegas showgirl, but that was okay because I didn't look like a patient.

It was great to see my family. I could see their worry, but I wore my wig to the wedding and was glad to see everyone. The wedding and reception was my threshold for wearing the wig. By the time I had returned to the hotel, the wig was in my purse, and the buggy cap was back on my head. It was even more important that I was able to see my uncle Greg's wife, Pat. I knew that she had previous battles with cancer, but little did I know that this event would be the last time I would see her as she would have another cancer recurrence that would take her life. I got to see her and be surrounded by family. That meant more to me than anything.

This trip also taught me a thing or two about myself. Just because I am sick doesn't mean that I have to look sick. I learned some tricks to attempt to look normal. Even though it may seem superficial, seeing myself looking somewhat normal was good for me and my mental health. I didn't want to appear weak.

I did sometimes take things a little too far. Even my own father said that sometimes my fake eyelashes looked "cartoonish." What does he know? I looked in the mirror and didn't see the effects of cancer as strong. I bought stencils to do a variety of shapes of eyebrows and definitely incorporated the help of the teenagers in my house showing me YouTube makeup tutorials.

One moment that made me laugh was when I went back to work at school that fall. I was teaching a lesson to a class of fifth graders. I was walking around the class and engaging the students in the instruction when it happened. I had a hot flash! I got so overheated that it must have melted the glue holding my eyelashes on, and one fell off into one of the student's notebooks. Of course, everyone was paying attention and saw it happen. Silence . . . So I picked up my lash and ripped the other one off and stuck it to my laptop until later. Fifth graders always have something to say, but this time, watching their teacher have her eyelashes randomly fall off was just too much to handle and forced them all into silence. I just kept on teaching.

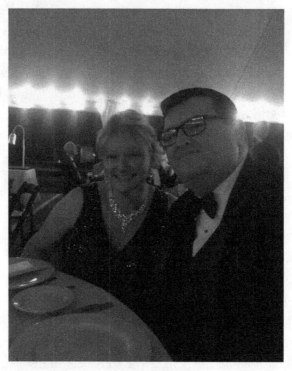

TJ and Becky attending the Riverside Shore Memorial Hospital Ball (Yes, that is a wig!)

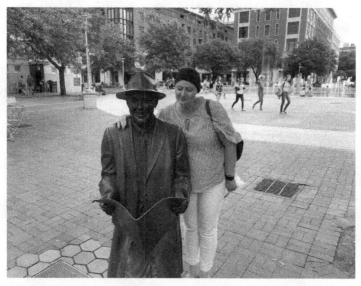

(Becky in Savannah, Georgia)

Chapter 12

Going through the Motions

I made it through those first four chemotherapies, and it was a rough time. I was bald, weak, and always tired. How much longer would this process go on? It seemed like forever. Now it was time for the weekly chemo. This time, I requested that my chemo schedule was changed from Fridays to Mondays. That whole chemo on Friday was messing up my weekend vibes. When I had chemo on a Monday, it gave me the opportunity to recuperate during the week and enjoy time with my family on the weekend.

Unfortunately, I was still weak and always nauseous, and feeling like this was more than I could handle. One of the things that got me through the hard days was positive thinking. Yes, that sounds cliché, but there is a lot of truth to that statement. I didn't always feel positive, and one moment that stuck with me through this whole journey was a conversation with TJ. TJ and I have been married for almost twenty years, and in that time, he never raised his voice to me until this one moment. We were sitting in the kitchen, and he was trying to get me to eat something. Everything tasted like metal and caused explosive sickness from both ends of my body.

"You have to eat. You are starving yourself," he pleaded.

I was laying my head on the kitchen island, turning away every suggestion he had. People were bringing us meals, but food was definitely the enemy to me. I knew I needed to eat, but I also knew the aftereffects of eating.

"Leave me alone, I just cannot eat. Even the smell of food is making me nauseous," I replied.

"I don't want to go to chemo anymore. I just want to end this and die. I cannot go on like this."

There was silence. I didn't see his face because my head was down on the island, but his voice thundered through me. TJ had a loud boisterous voice on a normal day. He was a high school football coach and a school administrator, so he knew how to raise his voice, and I don't think he ever understood the concept of a whisper.

"Damn it, Becky! Your ass is going to chemo each and every time the doctor tells you to be there. You are not leaving me with two teenage girls, your parents, and my mother to take care of. We are a team, and you cannot give up. I need you!" he yelled.

"I cannot do this much longer. I'm weak. I cannot even lift my head. Why am I doing this?" I answered.

"You are doing this because of your family. Be strong and get your shit together and go to chemo," he said.

That was the last time we ever talked about not making it through this. There was only a positive light on this after that rough conversation. I needed to hear from someone that giving up was not an option.

Once I was on the once-a-week treatments, things became a little better. I was still weak and dealing with nausea and diarrhea, but on a level of what I was experiencing with the first four treatments, this seemed all around better.

In June, three months into treatments, my daughter's schools were participating in the National Junior Beta Club competition in Savannah, Georgia. The girls were excited to participate and compete with their schools. TJ was planning to take the girls and be there to cheer them on. When I started talking about going, TJ was quick to shut me down that it would not be possible for me to travel for eight hours by car to Savannah. I had treatments to think about and how could I possibly handle a car ride for this long. My determined self insisted that I go on this trip. My chemo schedule had me leaving for Savannah the day after treatment and returning the day before the next treatment. I was not taking no for an answer. In my mind, I was keeping things normal for my children. I promised that I would rest and would even watch part of the convention on their Facebook Live event from the hotel room.

I made it to Savannah . . . barely. There were only a few moments that we had to do emergency bathroom stops. Those gas station restrooms would never be the same after I used them. After using the restrooms, I would run back to the car, wanting to leave like I had robbed the place.

We finally made it to Savannah, and that was when I realized that there was something else that I needed to face. In the lobby of the hotel were all the students from my school division's BETA teams. Most of them were my students who had not seen me since I mysteriously disappeared from work three months prior. How would they react? Would they recognize me? I wore my buggy cap on the ride and still had it on when I walked into the hotel lobby. Students whom I had spent every day with did not recognize me. They didn't figure it out until they noticed my daughters with me. Some of my students did not even know that I was sick. Not only was I sick, but also I looked worn out from an eight-hour car ride. I spent about an hour in the lobby of the hotel, getting hugs from my students. I felt so good to see them and not feel like I was hiding some deep secret. I packed my wig and never wore it. The kids saw me. They were comfortable, my own children were comfortable, and so was I.

I have absolutely no regrets going on that trip. Yes, I had some bad moments were I had to slow down or watch the convention virtually, but I cherish the good times of that trip. Dinners with friends, laughing, and feeling a bit normal. One thing about Savannah is it is known for being a haunted town. Madison and Morgan wanted to do a ghost tour, and since they were at the convention all day, it was my job to book a ghost tour. I went to the hotel lobby to see if the concierge had any suggestions for a reputable tour group. The concierge was excited to share one of the town's favorite ghost tours that tells you all about the ghosts of Savannah while riding around in a convertible funeral hearse. A funeral hearse . . . no, thank you. I quickly asked for other options as I had spent the last three months avoiding a funeral hearse in real life;

therefore, I was not going to pay and willingly get in one for a joyride around town. I ended up booking a ghost tour on a horse and carriage ride through the city. This was a much better situation. Morgan, who always loves a scary story, loved this trip, and seeing her joy brought me more joy than one could ever imagine.

I tried to make that summer normal, but as TJ would say, this was my new normal. Summertime to me always meant being by the water, whether it was at the beach, on a boat, or even by the pool. That was what my summers were like. My new normal had me having a skin reaction just walking out to the mailbox. The few times that I went out to enjoy a summer day, I was completely covered and under an umbrella. I was not enjoying this "new normal."

Another looming event was that in September, I would be having a double mastectomy. Once again, I advise staying away from online medical advice. Everyone is different, and using those types of platforms can make it worse for you. Just because a bunch of people in a Facebook group give medical advice, it does not mean you should listen to that instead of people who actually went to medical school. There were lots of scary things online about mastectomies. I consider myself young and want to feel and look good. Seeing pictures of women who had more stitch lines than Frankenstein and lots of scary scarring made me ponder what I would look like.

I needed something to take my mind off the surgery. Each year, the local hospital auxiliary has a ball to raise money for the local hospital. I had joined the auxiliary before my cancer diagnosis but did not do much, with the exception of sending in yearly dues and attending the ball each September. The ball was on a Saturday night, and my lymph node injection was planned for the following Monday afternoon, with surgery on Tuesday morning. TJ had questioned why we were even going. He quickly pointed out that it was a sit-down meal and I would eat toast and applesauce, it was open bar and I could not drink, and it was a lot of dancing and I could not even go upstairs without getting out of breath. I was determined to have a good time, and TJ humored me. It was a formal black-tie/gown event, so now I faced the whole looking-sick issue. Maybe I was making a mistake going out. I just felt like I needed one last hurrah before this surgery.

I had a gown that I could easily use the restroom in just in case. The next issue was my makeup and wig. Normally, I would have my long blonde hair in an updo or long and curled. Now all I had to work with was this wig. I made a makeup and a hair appointment with the ladies who normally cut my hair. I imagine that they probably were a bit mystified on why the bald woman made a hair appointment, but I had a plan.

On the day of the ball, I showed up to my hairstylist with the wig. "What can you do with this?" I asked.

My young stylist, Hartley, was actually excited by the challenge. She looked at me and looked at the wig and then back at me.

"I have ideas," she replied.

I let her have creative rights on whatever she could do to make a wig that usually spent time in my purse look like something elegant. She brushed it, shook it a couple of times, and placed it on my head and got to work. By the time she finished, it was clear that she had completed a Jesus-level miracle. She got to work on my makeup, and I brought her some super glam lashes. When she finished and turned the chair around, I didn't recognize the person sitting there. I was so excited and couldn't wait to show TJ who he was taking to the ball tonight.

When I arrived, people didn't recognize me. One person even admitted that when they saw me, they thought TJ was stepping out with another woman. I laughed because it was just me in a dolled-up wig and lashes. The true test was when my oncologist, Dr. Laura, walked in with her husband. Now remember, this is a woman that I see every week for the past six months. I said hello, and she said hello in return and kept walking. Then suddenly, she stopped in her tracks, turned, and looked at me carefully. Her face lit up when she realized that this was not some strange woman she didn't know saying hello. This was a strange woman whom she had to deal with every week. We laughed at how she didn't recognize me. I told her husband about how she couldn't tell him about me, but nothing was stopping me, and how I was her favorite patient and how she saved my life. It was a great moment to spend time with her outside of the cancer center setting.

Was TJ right about me not being able to party like in the past? Yes, he was absolutely correct. I tried to dance and have fun but would catch myself out of breath, needing to sit down. Finally, TJ said that I proved my point, and it was time to go home. The moment I sat in the car for the ride home, I took my wig off and flung it on the back seat of the car. The look on the valet parking attendant was priceless when he watched me remove the wig without care.

Chapter 13

Demolition Day

My weekend had ended, and now it was time to face the music. It was time for the mastectomy and moving forward in this process. Part of me was excited because this means that I was a little bit closer to the finish line. Another part of me was looking in the mirror at my bare breasts, knowing that today was their last day on my body. Before the demolition started, I had to do a lymphatic mapping with a sentinel node biopsy. The sentinel nodes are the first lymph nodes that a tumor drains into. By doing the mapping, a doctor injects a tracer material so that during the mastectomy, the lymph nodes can be located and removed. Once removed, they each go through further biopsy. This shows whether my past chemotherapies have been working or not.

Since several of my friends had been through this procedure, I felt that it was necessary to know everything about their experience. One friend told me that the injection was extremely painful and that she felt like she was "coming out of her skin." Another friend said it was just like any injection and no big deal. They each went to different hospitals to have this procedure done, and neither of their hospitals were the same that I would be going to have it done. Now my mind is clouded with the what-ifs of this procedure.

I asked Dr. Jenny about the injection, and she said that it was easy compared to everything I have been through. Was she just telling me that so I don't slip out the back door and run away? She had never been one to sugarcoat anything in this process, so why should I expect that now?

Since the surgery was going to be in a hospital an hour and a half away from my home and I had to have the lymph node injection the afternoon before the surgery, TJ and I decided that we would stay at a hotel near the hospital. This way, we didn't have to battle traffic on the way to the surgical center early in the morning.

The first task to be completed was the injection. I think that I was more nervous about that than the mastectomy. We arrived at the hospital on Monday afternoon, and it seemed as if it was forever before I was taken back. Finally, I was called back and led down a maze of hallways to a room with an examination table and what seemed like the makings of a mad scientist's lab. There were all kinds of equipment. TJ was allowed back with me, but they remanded him to a small hallway waiting area. The nurse was a kind, young gentleman, who was busy preparing all the materials for the doctor. Of course, I was quizzing him about the process and how bad it would hurt. He told me that it would be over before I knew it. That did not answer my question and certainly did not give me peace of mind.

The doctor came in and started to explain the procedure. My mind was a mess with worry. I only heard half of what he said. It was obvious that he could sense my anxiety, so he told a joke. I don't remember the exact joke, but I do recall that it would be classified in the category of a "dad joke." My nervousness triggered a laugh, even though he had already started with me and I felt a slight sting in my left breast area. I was waiting for the intense pain. The doctor said, "All done."

"What? That's it?" I responded, surprised.

"Yes, Mrs. Johnson, I tell a joke, you laugh, and I am done. It can be a painful experience, but we use a local injection to reduce the level of pain. You obviously were worried for nothing."

I was worried for nothing. It ached a little after the local anesthetic wore off, but it was nowhere near the big, scary thoughts that were occupying my head. Now I had to mentally prepare myself for the next step: the double mastectomy. TJ and I went out for dinner. We held hands through dinner and talked about all the things we had been through over the years. It was a time of reflection, the good times and the bad. One thing that was consistent was that we made it through, and we would make it through this as well. Once we checked into the hotel, it was time to go to bed because 5:00 a.m. will be upon us quickly. TJ has always had a knack of falling instantly asleep. He puts his head to the pillow, and the next thing I know, he is snoring. I, on the other hand, have to toss, turn, look at my phone, toss and turn some more, flip the pillow, and kick the blankets this way and that before I can properly fall asleep. Now I not only have my routine but also have thoughts of an impending surgery in the morning. I finally fell asleep, but the alarm going off felt like I had five minutes of sleep. I had a checklist of things to do before arriving at the surgical center. First was to not take any food or drink starting at midnight, and second was to take a shower the morning of the surgery using a surgical soap. I also had a bag packed with a special surgical bra from the plastic surgeon. I was told to make sure that this bra went with me into surgery as the doctor would put it on me at the end of the surgery. I also had pajamas that button on the front as I would not be able to lift my arms for a T-shirt type of top. It was the moment of truth.

We arrived at the surgical center and saw that I was in the first group of surgeries for the morning. Check-in was no different than any other time I have had a surgical procedure, except this time, I would have to spend the night at the hospital. All my other surgeries were small outpatient procedures. I was taken back to a small room, and everything was laid out for me. There was a hospital gown, those terrible "no slip" socks that don't fit anyone, and a paper bag for my belongings. I changed and got on the bed and waited.

"Hey, honey bunny, you ready for this?" Dr. Jenny said as she entered the room.

Is anyone ever ready for this? Her enthusiasm made me lie to her and tell her that I was ready. She went over everything again. The first breast would be removed, and once she moved to the other side, Dr. Teddy would come in to place the tissue expander. He would finish the surgery as he would place the tissue expanders on both sides. They were a good team and had this routine down to a science. TJ was also brought back, and Dr. Jenny explained how long the surgery would take and how I would be brought back to this room for recovery and then sent over to the main hospital for the evening. Before I knew what was happening, an IV was put in my hand, and the anesthesiologist had arrived to review his process. I knew it was protocol to review with a patient every step they would complete, but in my mind, I didn't care. He could have said that he was going to inject Kool Aid in my veins, and I would not have heard it. I just wanted to go to sleep and get this over with. TJ told me that he was going to slip out for a short while to get breakfast and he would be back quickly. I don't remember much more because the anesthesiologist had started injecting what I called the "sleepy time" medicine into the IV. It was another instance of me not remembering entering the operating room. I remember the chatter of the nurses wheeling me down the hall, but it sounded so distant. I remember the lights on the ceiling, and everything went dark.

I woke up back in the original room. Everything was blurry, and the sound of everyone's voices sounded so far away. TJ was sitting there, and someone was telling him that it went well. That person then addressed me. They were chipper and telling me that I did great. I was so drained and tired that I just drifted back out again.

I recall being moved from the surgical center to the main hospital. I was coherent enough to know that I was being moved, but not enough to figure out where I was or where I was going. I heard someone say to me to rest and everything was okay. So that was what I did, and I closed my eyes.

As the anesthesia started to wear off, my vision was still a little blurry, and my hearing sounded more like an echo. I heard a voice calling my name.

"Mrs. Johnson, you did great. How are you feeling?"

I opened my eyes to see a man, a man who looked very similar to the actor Joe Manganiello. If you are not familiar with this actor, he played a role in the movie *Magic Mike*, a story about male exotic dancers. In my messed-up mind, I thought that I may have died, and Joe Manganiello was welcoming me to heaven.

Then my Joe look-alike said, "Your husband is bringing up your bags from the car and will be here in a few minutes."

Reality struck as I was very much alive, and this was not Joe Manganiello in scrubs. This very handsome gentleman was my nurse. There I was drooling on myself and in my bald glory because my buggy cap was missing. TJ rushed in as Nurse Joe (as I secretly called him) was explaining how important it was for me to go to the bathroom soon and how he would help me. Nurse Joe was more than just eye candy. He was constantly checking on me and waking me up for blood pressure checks and helping me to the restroom. Nurse Joe was a bit of a task master with a handsome façade.

My friend Krysten and her husband, Chuck, came to visit me shortly after being put into the hospital room. I was still groggy and blissfully unaware of what was underneath the bandages. I could barely even move to see the bandages, let alone to know what was under them. I was in a fog, so I knew that they were talking to TJ and something about dinner. Food was the last thing on my mind, and I could also hear bits and pieces of discussion of me. The next thing I knew, I was all alone. Everyone had left to go home for the evening. Even Nurse Joe left. The new nurse wrote her name on the little whiteboard in the hospital room and did all the checks that Nurse Joe had completed. I started to drift away into sleep.

The first time it happened was early in the evening. When I heard it, I thought I was dreaming. It was a lullaby playing. The nurse came in to do her routine checks, and I told her that I think I heard a lullaby or maybe that was just in my head. She laughed and reassured me that I did hear a lullaby and it was not me hallucinating. The hospital had a tradition for every time a baby is born in the maternity ward, the hospital plays a lullaby over the loudspeaker. I smiled because this was the same hospital where both of my daughters were born, and I was flooded with memories of the exciting times of their births. My eyes flooded up with some sadness and some joy. I thought about the families on the maternity ward rejoicing over their new child. I wished to return to those moments of everyone being excited for a new little precious life. Now I was here for the fight of my life, trying to stop the ugly face of cancer so I can remain with my family.

The first time the lullaby woke me from my groggy slumber was endearing. By the seventh time, I was irritated and wondering why everyone decided to have a baby on the night I spend at the hospital. Between the nonstop birthing of babies and the nurses coming in to check me out and see if I need to use the restroom, I got no sleep. The best sleep I got was when I was on the operation table. I did fall asleep to get about a half hour of sleep, only to awaken at 5:00 a.m. by Dr. Teddy. He does patient rounds early. Does this man even sleep? It was five in the morning, and he looked chipper and happy. He proceeded to check under the bandages and praise his work. He told me everything I needed to know about my recovery at home. He talked about the three drains that I had and how they need to be emptied and the blood amounts recorded. Also, he talked about keeping that ugly surgical bra that he gave me on. To this day, I still wear the ugly plastic surgery bra. I have purchased more from Amazon because I wore them so much that the eye hooks fell off. Before surgery, all my follow-up appointments were made so that there would be no confusion on when I would return to his office. He told me that Dr. Jenny would stop by and would complete the release paperwork so that I could go home today and that he had sent my prescriptions to the hospital pharmacy, so I needed to pick them up before discharge. I just nodded my head as if I were listening, and he left in his chipper glory to go wake up another patient.

I lay in the bed, listening to all the hospital noises. The staff shifts were changing, and Nurse Joe was back.

"Did you have a restful night?" he asked.

I think the look on my face told the story. I gave him the abbreviated version of my evening with all the babies born, nurse visits, and Dr. Teddy's 5:00 a.m. wake up call. The good part was that I would be released today into the wild. It was exciting knowing that I was going home to rest in my own bed without the noise of the hospital. I would gratefully accept the noise of my family.

My next visitor was Dr. Jenny making her patient rounds. She checked under the bandages and repeated all of the same rules that Dr. Teddy gave me. This was good because I was certainly a groggy mess the first time the directions were given. She also had a Ziploc bag in her hand that had folded material in it.

"This is for you. My mother makes these for me to give to all of my patients. It's a little cami top that has pockets for the drains to fit into," Dr. Jenny said as she handed me the bag.

Little did I know that this item was as valuable as gold. It was something that I stayed in the entire time of my recovery with the drains. It was so amazing that my mother even used it as a pattern to make the same cami top for some ladies that I knew locally who were going through the same operation with drains. It was perfect for wearing under pajamas, but with hot flashes from the chemo, I was wearing only this cami top all day, every day. The pockets on the inside were perfect for holding the drains. The drains are little clear plastic grenade-like things that had a long tube inside the incision. "During a mastectomy, the breast is separated from subcutaneous tissue and muscle. This results in a raw surface that leaks fluid called serous fluid. Although serous fluid production is normal, we don't want the fluid to stay inside, we want it to come out, so a drain is placed." (https://www. breastinstitutehouston.com/post-mastectomy-wound-care/)

I had three of these lovely drains. My left side had two, and my right side had one. Every twelve hours, the drains needed to be emptied, and the line to the incision needed to be cleared. Nurse Joe called it "threading the line." He showed me how to do it, and Dr. Teddy left a chart for me to complete at home with the measurements of this serous fluid that just looked like really clotted blood. There was also a technique of squeezing the drain and then capping it shut so that there was no air inside. TJ walked in at the end of the drain upkeep lesson and was quick to turn around and walk back to the hallway. This was a solid no from him on helping do this. He would feel faint just looking at the drains, not even getting to the process of emptying them. I figured that I could call on my mother-in-law, who is a nurse, to come over, but that would be a lot to ask, especially since it was twice a day. I could try to get someone at my own residence to do it. My dad was an option because he would always help when the girls would have a loose tooth. He didn't get squeamish around that, so he should be able to handle this. Madison was also an option since she wanted to go into premed. TJ was definitely not an option.

Once the drain tutorial was finished, I was discharged to go home. TJ was sent to get my prescriptions and bring the car around to the front of the hospital. Nurse Joe was going to wheel me down to the car. Down the elevator I went, and when the doors opened to the hospital front lobby, I heard something. It was classical piano music. As I entered the lobby, a roar of applause came from a crowd that had gathered. *For me?* I thought. No, Nurse Joe informed me that a donor to the hospital sent a classical pianist to the hospital to play the baby grand piano in the lobby once a week for all to enjoy. Even though it wasn't for me, it gave me a few minutes to enjoy the fanfare as if it were for me. It was the perfect send-off from this part of the journey.

The ride home seemed fast, but I did feel every bump and pothole on the highway home. Now it was time to recover. I still had not seen what was hidden beneath the bandages, but all the doctors who looked seemed satisfied with the results. The true test was whether or not I could handle seeing the results. That moment came fast. I was able to take a shower and had come out of the cami top. The hospital gave me this plastic string that made me able to wear the drains like a necklace. I stood in front of the full-length mirror in my bathroom. It was not as bad as I anticipated, but it was certainly a lot to take in.

The stitches were there like perfect letter U's under each breast. The nipples were gone. Did this mean I could go topless? When you think about it, the purpose of tops, such as a bikini top, is to cover the nipples. Now that they are gone, what is stopping me from going wild and free? I knew what was stopping me. It was the absolute horror that others would have looking at this. It was depressing. When the swelling and the bruising leave, what will it look like?

I had about a month to recover before starting the radiation treatment. During that time, I would be getting what I called "fill-ups" from the plastic surgeon. In each tissue expander, there was a port.

The doctor would access it by using a magnet to find the port and then injecting saline to stretch the skin and increase the size of the breast gradually. I went once a week for these fill-ups. The radiologist warned me not to "overfill" the expanders because it could block the radiation to certain areas. I didn't want overly large breasts for my new look. TJ, on the other hand, had encouraging words for extra saline in the expanders. Unfortunately for him, I had to follow the doctor's orders.

The first time I went for a fill-up, I had nervous jitters. Of course, my mind went instantly to how bad it was going to hurt. Yes, I am a wimp when it comes to pain, and I don't like surprises. I was sitting in the paper vest when Dr. Teddy came into the room for the first injections. During the surgery, I already had a small amount of saline in the tissue expanders. I would get a syringe full on each side. As he prepped the area for the first injection, he had a magnet on a chain. The magnet attached to the port, and he marked it with a Sharpie marker. Here I was again, feeling faint. I told Dr. Teddy that I wanted to lie down and that I was feeling nauseous and weak. He didn't miss a beat. He unwrapped an alcohol swab and put it on the bridge of my nose and told me to breath. It was a technique that had never been used on me. I was not sure if it actually stopped me from fainting or he just used that as a way to distract me, but it worked. He injected saline into the port, and I didn't feel a thing. It didn't pinch or even sting. Thanks to the mastectomy, I had no feeling in the breast area. I closed my eyes, and before I knew it, it was over. I had several more appointments like this, each time watching my breast size grow a little more.

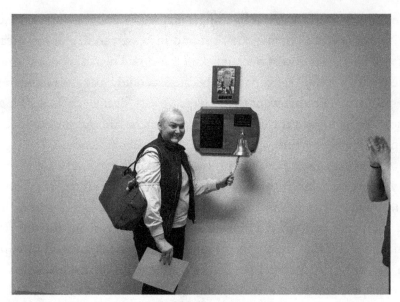

At the Riverside Cancer Center ringing the
bell for completion of Radiation.

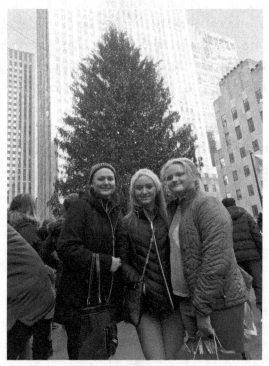

(Becky, Madison and Morgan at Rockefeller Center at Christmas)

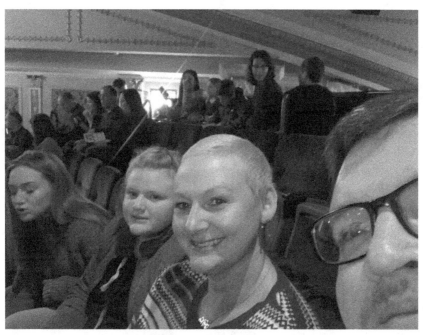

(School of Rock on Broadway Left to Right
Madison, Morgan, Becky and TJ)

Chapter 14

Simply Glowing

When one is facing radiation treatment, it is not wise to watch documentaries on the Chernobyl accident. I was facing twenty-five radiation treatments, and I had finished watching a series on the effects of a radiation accident on a Russian town. Yes, not my best decision. I knew that this would not be a catastrophic event like Chernobyl and that people did this treatment every day, but it was still scary. The radiologist sent me for "marking" to prepare for how the radiation machine would be set for my daily visit. It was basically an MRI. Some people get actual tattoo dots to show the marks for where the radiation should be directed. I didn't need a tattoo, even though I was secretly hoping that I would since it would be my first tattoo. I guess one cannot claim to be a badass with a freckle as a tattoo.

Within a week, my radiation treatment schedule was set. I started at the end of November, and my final treatment was December 23. This was going to be a radioactive Christmas. I thought that I had everything figured out. Being a mom, you automatically get the skill of using every second wisely. I had returned to work and snagged the last radiation appointment of the day. Therefore, I could leave school and go directly to the radiation, get zapped, and go home to dinner, homework, and general catching up around the house. The thing that I didn't understand was that even though I would lie in the radiation machine and let it do its thing, it was exhausting. Not only was it zapping cancer, but it was zapping my energy as well. I would come home like a zombie. Up the stairs I would go and fall asleep. It took everything I had to eat something and shower.

Going to radiation each day was an easy process. I was given a card that I scanned when I walked in. It was like a Disney easy pass but for radiation. The cancer center had a little changing room to keep my things and put on a hospital gown top. In the radiation room, there were cubbies for each patient if they required extra equipment. Of course, I required extra equipment. I had a gel-like mat that would intensify the radiation on the area that it was placed. This mat would only be used for about ten sessions, and it was only placed on my left breast. When it was placed on me, it was freezing cold, but it didn't stay that way for long. The radiation techs would start by making sure the marks that were drawn on my skin were matching with the machine. Sometimes, the alignment would be changed, and new marks were made.

At first, I thought this was relatively easy. I go in, lie down, and stay still in the position that the techs place me in. The hard part in the beginning was being able to keep my arms above my head. From the mastectomy, it was very difficult to have a full range of motion of my arms, particularly the left arm, because of the removal of the lymph nodes. Dr. Jenny knew that this would be an issue before I even started the radiation. She had already set up physical therapy appointments prior to me starting the radiation. Physical therapy after a mastectomy can be physically draining, but it is worth being able to have as much range of motion back as possible. I was already struggling to lift my arms, and then the situation was compounded with the radiation shrinking the skin affected. Luckily, the physical therapy did exactly what was needed for me to lift my arms for the radiation treatment.

The deeper I ventured into treatment, the more I realized that this would not be a mere walk in the park. I was prescribed a silver sulfadiazine, known as Silvadene cream, for the treatment of burns. It didn't become real to me until one day, I was lying there and I could smell something burning. The reality was that it was me burning. Each day, I looked in the mirror to see burns and peeling skin. I would slather the prescription cream on my breasts, hoping that it would take the pain away. I was prescribed pain medication again, which I only took in the evening so I could actually sleep. I didn't like pain medication because I don't like the feeling of being out of control, but in this situation, it was critical to being able to sleep. My left breast was a bright red, and TJ would say that he could feel the heat from the burns coming through my shirt.

I think that it is a good rule of thumb for people to mind their business when seeing someone who may be going through a treatment unless you want to offer words of encouragement. It was amazing how many people would see that glowing red that reached as high as the left side of my neck and would make an unnecessary comment. One day after radiation, I stopped at a convenience store, and in line, a woman said, "You need to stay out of the sun. Cancer is in your future." I have always had difficulty holding my tongue, and this time was no different. My response was as follows:

"Cancer is in the present for me because this is not sunburn but radiation treatment burns. I am a cancer survivor, so mind your business."

The woman was taken by surprise and walked out the door without anything to say. The cashier looked at me, nodding her head, and said, "That is right. Preach it."

I walked out with my head held high, but even though hair was starting to sprout on my head, the burns continued to make me a face of cancer.

I finished radiation treatment on December 23, 2019. I ran the bell at the cancer center to symbolize the completion of treatment. Unfortunately, the ringing of the bell was premature. There were some setbacks in my future, but at this moment, I was overwhelmed with joy that I rang that bell like a manic.

TJ and I decided that we needed to do something to celebrate this milestone in my treatment. We also felt that it would be good for our entire family's mental health to get away for a trip. I had been very worried about how my daughters were handling the roller-coaster ride of my treatment, so we definitely needed a time to be together, not talking about cancer, not talking about doctors, and definitely not talking about the pain. Morgan had thrown herself into being part of the local theater group, and this was a positive way for her to cope with all the things that were happening to our family. The group at the theater welcomed her with open arms, and being there gave her joy. So it was not surprising that for Christmas, she asked to go to New York City to see a Broadway show. TJ and I discussed making this a day-after-Christmas trip. We would take the Amtrak train into the city, stay for several nights, see a show, and enjoy a New York City Christmas.

The plan was in motion, and we would see the show *School of Rock*. I was probably not in the best physical state for this trip, but I was determined to have an amazing family outing and bring some level of normalcy back to our lives. Even though my burns were severe and I was in pain, I was determined to make this an unforgettable moment.

We took the Amtrak into the city and had a small apartment that was near Times Square. Everywhere we wanted to go was within walking distance. Yes, physically, my body was struggling and I was weak, but this was exactly what I needed mentally. Seeing the smiles on my daughters' faces and hearing their laughter brought so much joy to me. This was what I needed. Often, I wondered how I was able to keep up, and I really don't know how, but it is definitely one of my favorite times with my family.

The first night we had dinner at Tavern on the Green. New York City was still in the Christmas spirit. The Macy's window was decorated, and the sidewalk in front of the windows was shoulder to shoulder of people. As I walked through Times Square, my mind wasn't on the lights and excitement, but on constantly making sure that someone on the busy streets didn't bump into me. At this point, not only was I burned, but also I was blistered. The streets were bustling, and I felt like Madison and Morgan were watching over me like a nervous parent instead of vice versa.

My appetite was limited, and I didn't want to be sick from eating, which seemed to rule my entire life. Even though my physical condition was limited, it didn't stop me from enjoying everything and everyone around me. Part of me felt that I was now looking at life differently.

If I weren't going through cancer, would my perspective of this trip be different? I had always been a rigid schedule planner and would be upset if anything changed my plans. This time, I was more of a free spirit who was just enjoying the ride.

Speaking of enjoying the ride, on the second evening, we went to see *School of Rock* on Broadway. Watching Morgan sitting on the edge of her seat, taking everything in, was just as exciting as watching the show. It had been one of the toughest years our family had ever experienced, so it was a relief to have us all together in such an upbeat, happy atmosphere. When the show ended, we would have to walk several blocks back to the apartment. I was drained, and TJ was able to read the cues that I was giving off. He started looking for a taxi to take us back, but everything was taken. He was starting to look frustrated as two men on bicycles pedaled up to us. They had carriages attached to their bikes. It was called a pedicab, but it reminded me of a rickshaw. TJ and Madison climbed into one, and Morgan and I climbed into another. The drivers had thought of everything. They gave us each a blanket to stay warm and played Frank Sinatra's song *New York, New York* on their iPhones.

This was great, I thought as we pulled into traffic. Then I realized that pedicabs are the equivalent of a roller-coaster ride. We were dodging cars and people. At times, we were so close to traffic that I could reach my hand out of the carriage and touch the vehicle next to us. Morgan and I just held each other tight, laughing, watching reactions from the pedestrians and drivers. We noticed that TJ and Madison were doing the same. We certainly saw the city in a way that I had not expected. When we arrived at the apartment, we were all a bit shaken. The girls were laughing and ran ahead of TJ and I past the doorman into the apartment building. TJ and I seemed to hold each other up, walking in.

"Cancer cannot kill me, but a pedicab in New York City may." I laughed.

TJ laughed and said that it was the most expensive and dangerous bicycle ride he had ever had in his life.

Chapter 15

Two Steps Forward, Three Steps Back

My radioactive Christmas was over, and I had to face the music of my lymph node pathology report. I knew shortly after the mastectomy that several of my lymph nodes came back positive. This was hard information to take since I felt like everything was moving in the right direction. I did everything I was told to do, and the cancer was still there. All the doctors on my team had the same concerns since I was high risk for recurrence and a clinical stage 3 without a full response to neoadjuvant therapy. In layman's terms, I still have cancer. All that chemotherapy and radiation and I still have cancer.

A plan was developed for me to continue chemotherapy from January to the end of October using a chemo called ado-trastuzumab (Kadcyla). This bump in the road would delay the transfer of the tissue expanders to breast implants. Here I thought I was at the finish line, and now the line was moved further.

I was taking different medications that were messing with my hormonal balance. My mood was changing, and I even noticed myself becoming a little more aggressive and assertive in behavior. I was taking a pill called anastrozole. This is a hormone-based chemotherapy pill that is a nonsteroidal aromatase inhibitor. It decreases the amount of estrogen that I would make. I was also getting a Trelstar shot every twelve weeks. This injection is a hormone therapy that is normally used for prostate cancer. It has also shown positive results with my type of breast cancer. TJ was starting to get concerned with my mood swings. It was becoming more than a little hormonal. I had three events that led to TJ speaking up at one of my oncology checkups.

The first time was me waiting in line at the Walmart checkout. I was tired and having hot flashes, and I always seemed to end up in the line that "has a problem." The cashier was a patient older lady who was dealing with a lady using coupons. The coupons were not scanning correctly. At this point, I was fanning myself with a tabloid magazine and leaning on the conveyer. TJ offered to take care of this, handing me the keys to go wait in the car, but I refused. My stubbornness had me thinking that I could make this go faster. The cashier called the floor manager, Eddie. I remember him walking toward our checkout and then walking past it to several rows down. He was having a casual conversation with a young checker and seemed to dismiss the need at my checkout. I looked at our cashier. Was she going to do something? It seemed as if an eternity had passed as she said nothing. I felt that this was my cue to step in and help. So I yelled, "Hey, Eddie, you are kind of needed over here." TJ was mortified. He said the Walmart got so quiet, you could have heard a mouse fart. Eddie was also a bit caught off guard. He turned bright red and ran over to the register to handle the coupon catastrophe going on at our checkout. When it was my turn to check out, Eddie scampered away as quickly as he arrived. The sweet cashier went, "How do you know Eddie?"

My response was rude and unwarranted. "I don't know Eddie. I read it off his name tag. I, unlike you, am not intimidated by a teenager in a Walmart smock."

I walked away, pushing the cart. TJ was beyond irritated with me. How could I be so rude to such a sweet little older lady? In retrospect, I am definitely embarrassed by my behavior. I had a habit of being sassy at times, but I was never like this.

The second incident happened when I picked up my oldest from sports practice. I was sitting in my car, waiting for Madison to come out, and one of the groundskeepers was starting up a weed whacker. The noise of the machine got my attention because I noticed that the man was right next to my car, throwing grass and stones all around. I felt my blood boil. I hopped out of my car and grabbed the machine.

"What are you doing? You are throwing stuff on my car! Where is your car? Let's see how much you like it!" I yelled.

The man seemed shocked, but not necessarily apologetic. He took the weed whacker back and decided to do this far away from me.

The third incident was what TJ said was the "straw that broke the camel's back" on my behavior.

I had stopped at a convenience store after chemo and walked out to see a man intently looking into my car. Was this man trying to break into my car in broad daylight in front of a busy convenience store? I yelled, "Hey, is there something in my car that belongs to you?" I had surprised this man to the point that he grabbed at his chest.

"Ma'am, I am so sorry. My wife and I are looking at this type of car, and we have narrowed it down to this and another type. I walked by and noticed it. I am sorry," he said.

There was silence. Everyone in the parking lot had to stop to see what was going to happen. I had not thought this all the way through. If he was stealing my car, what was I going to do? What if he had a gun? Fortunately for me, he actually was just looking at the car and not planning to steal it. I felt bad and showed him all the cool features of my car and then sent him on his way with a stern warning. "Don't do that again. You don't know what kind of crazy person you will come across." He nodded and apologized again.

When I broke down and told TJ, he was furious at me. "You could have been killed. Cancer is not going to kill you. Your mouth is going to get you shot." At my next oncology appointment, he told Dr. Laura his concerns. It was decided from that point on to stop the anastrozole and Trelstar. TJ felt that taking me off that medicine was a community service to all.

It seemed that once off those medications, I was not as bad of a behavior issue. I was still receiving the chemotherapy but was excited that the ado-trastuzumab (Kadcyla) did not cause hair loss. I was actually getting some hair growing on my head. The problem was that

I really did not remember what my actual hair color was because as a child, I was a blonde; in my teens, my hair was darker; and before chemotherapy, I was blonde. Now the hair was coming back, and it didn't come back blonde or brown. It came back, as TJ called it, calico. I had brown patches, gray patches, blondish patches, and the like. I still wore my buggy cap, but it was more to cover the crazy hair that was coming in at about a half inch long. It was time to take care of that. Even though I probably shouldn't have been running to get my hair dyed, I did it anyway. I went to my usual ladies who have proven to be experts in beautifying an old lady with cancer. I wanted to do something wild and different. The plan in my head was bright blonde. When the chair turned around, I loved it. It was different and a little bit of a rocker look. This was the new me. TJ said that I needed to embrace my new normal, so why not make my normal a little rock star–like.

Chapter 16

What Happens in Vegas . . .

Technically, this chapter should say I went to Vegas, and that was the end of the story. With my new rocker hair and a zest to embrace life, I started to check things off my imagined bucket list. Basically, as things came up, I jumped with the enthusiasm of someone with limited time. I had always wanted to see Jimmy Buffett, live and when he was playing at a nearby concert, I was all on board for that good time. I told TJ that I wanted to see him live before he or I died. We checked that off the list, but the biggest adventure was yet to come.

We are friends with a couple who has been dating for several years, Rodger and Michelle. Rodger had pulled TJ aside one day and said that he planned to ask Michelle to marry him on her birthday. The catch was that he wanted to pop the question in front of the fountain at the Bellagio Hotel in Las Vegas. Rodger asked if we wanted to come along. TJ was worried. Could I handle such a trip? I had done day trips, but nothing so far. Rodger was one who always had surprises up his sleeves and had made arrangements to see Aerosmith live. When TJ presented this idea, I was excited. Of course, TJ was more worried that I could not handle so much activity.

I wanted to see my friends get engaged. It was an amazing moment to share with them. Plus, I was never allowed by my parents to see Aerosmith as a teen. My dad said that they did not follow our family values and that the atmosphere of the concert was not appropriate for me as a teen. Now, in my forties, I wanted to be corrupted by attending an Aerosmith concert and what better place than Las Vegas.

There were some things that I would have to bring on this trip other than some cool Vegas clothes. I had to bring compression arm sleeves that were now a daily part of my life. Without lymph nodes on my left side, I started to have fluid buildup and difficulty with range of motion in that arm. I had three compression sleeves. The first one was a plain skin-tone sleeve with high compression. This was to be worn when I had a high level of fluid buildup. It was also used when you were sedentary for a long period of time. It was important to wear this device on the plane since I would be sitting for over seven hours and the air compression in the plane may cause issues. The second sleeve had a medium level of compression. I was able to get this one in colors and designs. Of course, I ordered it to look like a sleeve of tattoos. If I am going to have to wear it, I should have some fun with it. I certainly got a lot of comments on it. People I knew forever would say things like "I never knew you had tattoos," and people I didn't know had their eyes instantly drawn to it. It was fun for a medical garment and would probably go along with my Vegas look. The third sleeve was unfortunately the least cool of all three pieces. It was a sleeping sleeve. It looked like a giant oven mitt that went all the way up the arm. This sleeve was hot and uncomfortable, and I couldn't sleep when I wear it. Most of the time, it would end up on the floor next to my bed because it was so unbearable.

The big item that had to make this journey was a lymphedema pump. Nothing screams "I am so uncool" than a medical device that gets you handicap seating on the plane. A way to treat lymphedema, aside from the compression sleeves, is the use of manual massage. Because of the severity of my lymphedema, I was eligible for a pump. In my mind, it was another sleeve, but this one compressed very similar to what a physical therapist would do to manually push the fluid out of my arm. My imagination and what actually arrived for me were two different things. The company that sends out this machine to patients was extremely efficient. They even sent a representative to my home on a Sunday, on a holiday weekend. This pump was more than just an electronic compression sleeve. It was a pump with long hoses, the hoses connected to a duo of pieces. The first piece was a sleeve that wrapped around the waist and Velcros shut. It resembled a one-arm straitjacket. The second piece was a pair of shorts. My initial reaction was that the representative brought the wrong machine because my issue was in my left arm, not in my waist or legs. This was when I learned that when the fluid is moved out of the arm, it goes to other places, and this suit helps to direct the fluid to other areas of the body with lymph nodes. The representative helped me get in the suit and showed me how my time in this suit was already preprogrammed into the pump. After she left, TJ was standing there, smirking. He was quick to point out that I looked like the Michelin Man in this suit. This was to be my routine for one hour each evening. Therefore, this lovely machine was going to Sin City as well. I had it packed in a duffel bag with all the pump paperwork that I was supposed to carry to board a plane.

My anxiety of carrying this machine with me was high. It was bulky and looked like something that would probably prompt security to stop me. I guess that airport security was well versed on lymphedema pumps because no one questioned this machine and why I had it. As a matter of fact, the flight staff took it and put it safely away and allowed me to board the plane first. TJ and I sat down in the plane and waited for the fun times to begin. Deep in my mind, I wondered if my arm would swell to Incredible Hulk size or if the swelling would even be noticeable.

I had more going on in my head than just making it through airport security with this device. Days before the trip, I had two appointments. The first was with the plastic surgeon. I would be having the tissue expanders and port removed, and breast implants would be put in. Also, I would be having more fat transfers. This is where the surgeon removes fat from my belly area to fill in areas around the implants to give a more natural look. I was all about fat removal and was quick to let the surgeon know that if he accidently removed too much fat, it was okay to dump the extra in the trash. It would not hurt my feelings. Unfortunately, the surgeon was not going to make some "tragic" mistake of removing too much belly fat.

The second big appointment was with the oncologist, Dr. Laura. Since I was officially finished with the chemotherapy treatments at the center, I was due for the next steps in the process. The plan was that I was to start one year of treatment of a medication called Nerlynx (neratinib). This medicine was approved in 2017 and was considered the first adjuvant therapy for woman with HER2 positive breast cancer. This medicine was special because it is a kinase inhibitor that blocks certain proteins in cancer cells. It keeps the cancer cells from dividing and greatly reduces the chances of cancer returning. Dr. Laura referred to this as targeted therapy. The big selling point of this medication was that after two years, 94 percent of the women taking this had no cancer recurrence.

I was overjoyed that this would be an opportunity for me and excited that I could possibly kick cancer's butt for the long term as well. It was decided that I would not start this medicine until after I returned from Vegas. There was a chance of diarrhea as a side effect, so it would be best to be home to see how my body reacts. Also, this was a medication that I could not receive at the local Walgreens. This medication had to come from a specialized pharmacy. It had to be shipped to my home, and someone had to sign for receiving the medicine. It also came with a price tag of a mere $18,000 a month. A lot of details had to be worked out with my health insurance before I possessed this miracle medicine. The plan was set that the day after I return from Vegas, I would start the regimen of six Nerlynx pills per day.

Like the saying "What happens in Vegas, stays in Vegas," there is not much to say. It was a wonderful time watching two friends get engaged. The trip was a welcomed distraction from all that had happened for the previous year and a half. Luckily, my lymphedema did not cause me to swell up like a tick, and for the most part, the side effects from my chemotherapy treatments were minimal. I came home in one of the healthiest mental states in a long time. I felt good. Looking out of the plane window, I wondered if I was turning a corner into feeling better.

Chapter 17

Satan's Medication

I came back from Vegas in probably the healthiest state of mind in a long time. I was officially finished with intravenous chemotherapy and was about to start the target therapy. This put me in a place in which I felt that the end of treatment was near. All I had left was a year of the Nerlynx and a surgery to transfer out the tissue expanders and replace them with breast implants. The finish line seemed to be in view.

Prior to my trip to Las Vegas, I had fielded several phone calls from the pharmacy that I would receive the Nerlynx. They were like nagging mothers calling every other day. They were full of questions. Had I received the medication? Had I started it? Did I know about the suggested diet for taking this medication? All these questions should have been a red flag to me. They even called me while I was sitting at a blackjack table in Vegas.

The second red flag should have been the dietary suggestions. I had to go through almost an hour training about eating while on this medicine. This was where I was introduced to the BRAT diet. This diet is a plethora of low-fiber, starchy, binding foods. The idea behind this diet is to make your stool firm and cut back on diarrhea and an upset stomach. BRAT stands for bananas, rice, applesauce, and toast. I was told that I could also incorporate crackers, chicken broth, oatmeal, and weak tea or flat soda. Eating was already a chore, and this was going to make it even more of a dreaded task than before. Another part of this medication was absolutely no alcohol. I have never been a big drinker but would enjoy a mixed drink every once in a while. It seemed that after I finished chemo, I craved the taste of a margarita. Just the smell of one was enough to throw me into orbit. The smell of the tequila was alluring in a way that it had never been before. I am not sure what changed to make me crave this so much. One night, TJ and I were at the local Mexican grill, and I even suggested ordering a margarita and just sticking my tongue in it and not drinking it. He just shook his head and laughed at me. Little did I know that this meal at the Mexican grill would be my last real meal before the entering the BRAT zone.

I started the Nerlynx pills on the day after returning from Vegas. Dr. Laura suggested that I take one on the first day, two on the second day, and so forth until I reached the daily dosage of six pills a day. I had small episodes of diarrhea, but nothing that caused me alarm. By the third day, in the afternoon, was when everything changed and not in a good way. I was at school, working in one of my last classes of the day, when it hit. The diarrhea hit, and it hit hard. Luckily, with my job, I worked with other teachers in the classroom, so I could exit quickly to pollute the restroom. I would like to take this moment to deeply apologize to everyone who used the faculty restroom after me. I tried everything, air freshener and Poo-Pourri, and nothing could take the terrible poo and sulfur-like metal smell out of the room. I was in and out of the classroom so much that the teacher I worked with was very concerned. I reassured her that everything was fine and it must have been something I ate. Little did I know that this would be my last day at work for quite a long time.

I had barely made it home from work. About two miles from my home, it hit. I was sweating, and my stomach was churning. I drove really fast, praying that I would not see the police officers who live in my neighborhood and praying that the deer that usually congregate in fields don't decide to do a suicide attempt with my car. I made it home. Barely. Our daughters both had things going on, and TJ and I had planned to go out to dinner. One whiff of our house and he was concerned if I should go or not. I told him that I was fine and that there was nothing left to exit my body. The plan for the evening was to go to one of our local Irish pubs for a romantic dinner for two. It was exciting, just the two of us. In my mind, I was going to eat the blandest thing that they had on the menu. Sitting in the pub and seeing the staff bring out food to everyone's table changed my mind. I cannot remember exactly what I ate, but I know it was not BRAT approved. Far from it! I do remember getting a side salad with my meal and TJ warning me that I probably should not eat it. I was deliriously hungry as everything I basically ate for the week was in the toilet at school. I ate with joy. It tasted wonderful. Then it hit! I was feeling the churning in my stomach. TJ, who was sitting across me in the noisy pub, said he could even hear it. I got up and walked as fast I could, trying to squeeze my buttocks tight, and gracefully walked to the restroom. In a small town, it is easy to know everyone in the restaurant. As I was quickly making my way to the back restroom, people were trying to stop me with "Hey, how are you?" I had no time to talk and quickly pushed through to the restroom. Luckily, it was empty. When I returned to the table, TJ had already paid the bill and was handing me my purse. He obviously did not want to stay at the scene of the poop crime.

In the car, he was reminding me that I should have stuck to the BRAT diet and I probably would not have polluted an Irish pub. He was right, but I didn't want to admit the error of my ways. Later, I would learn that BRAT diet or not, my body was going to have a severe battle with Nerlynx. Halfway home, it hit again, and we raced home. I made it home, but once again, barely. As the night progressed, I got worse. Now the diarrhea was not stopping. It was the equivalent of liquid lava rushing out of me. Plus, I got the added bonus of vomiting. By two in the morning, I was lying on the bathroom floor, shivering and hot. I no longer had food in my body, but I was still releasing what was probably bile. I was weak, and TJ panicked.

"I am taking you to the emergency room," TJ told me.

I didn't want to go, but at this point, I knew something was seriously wrong. This would be the first of many journeys to the local emergency room. TJ was always no-nonsense when it came to going to the hospital. His idea is if you need to go, you just get in the car and go. My idea is packing a bag, having all the medicines I take, having a spare pair of underwear, straightening my hair, and putting on some lipstick so I don't look dead. I was so weak that I couldn't even raise the hairbrush to my hair. I had a Ziploc bag to hold the vomit on the car ride and prayed that I would be able to clench my buttocks enough to make the fifteen-minute ride to the ER. My reason for trying not to look like I was on death's door was because I had taught for many years in the local public school system and it was inevitable that I would run into one of my past students. This was the same for TJ.

TJ raced in the ER to get me a wheelchair because at this point, I was too weak to get out of the car. The moment we rolled into the ER, the gentleman at the front desk called me by my maiden name. Of course, this gentleman was someone I taught in fourth grade at the beginning of my career. TJ also coached him in football. I was spotted out, in pajamas, smelling like vomit and poo. It seemed that getting recognized may have possibly given me some special treatment or they just didn't want to freak everyone out in the waiting room because I was taken directly back to a room in the emergency department.

One thing that Dr. Laura always reiterated to me was that if something happened and I found myself in the emergency room, I was always to identify myself as one of her patients immediately. It felt like I was in *Charlie and the Chocolate Factory* and had the golden ticket. I was definitely dehydrated and weak. The first thing that occurred was an IV was completed, and along with some fluids, anti-nausea medication was flowing. Once I got some fluids in me, I definitely started to feel better, but it would be a long night in the ER.

As I was lying there, listening to the click of the infusion machine, I started to hear the sounds of an unhappy patient. There was yelling of "No, no, no" coming from down the hall. It became more and more obvious that the person was someone who had some mental and emotional challenges. TJ and I had experienced these types of situations working in schools. This type of situation could escalate quickly. We heard the name Steve as the ER staff was trying to calm him down. He also had someone with him who was sort of a support monitor who was using de-escalation strategies. Suddenly, we heard Steve making a break for it and the staff calling for security. Apparently, Steve was a regular visitor to the emergency room as he was on a first-name basis with everyone, including security. Over the intercom, we heard, "Steve is on his way to the cafeteria." There was no description needed because everyone knew him. After gathering him up and returning him to the ER, he was still not compliant to the procedures that were going to take place. The noise started to get louder as it appeared that Steve was getting closer to our room. The room I was in had a sliding glass door with a curtain. The glass door was open, and we could hear clearly that Steve was making a break for it again, but this time, he grabbed scissors from one of the nurses. This was when Steve decided to threaten death by scissors to anyone getting close to him. TJ jumped up and quickly closed our glass door and held it shut so that we did not get a surprise visit from Steve and his stolen scissors. The situation came to a culmination with law enforcement tricking Steve out the scissors and him returning to a room. Later, as I was walking to the restroom with my IV machine, I passed Steve's room. He was in a bed and had several law enforcement officers with him. As I passed by, he yelled, "Hi, lady, I'm feeling better now." I just gave him a thumbs-up and carried on with my evening at the ER.

The next weekday, I had a follow-up appointment with Dr. Laura. It was decided that I would hold off on taking Nerlynx until after I had my implant transfer surgery in two weeks and had recovered. In my mind, I was relieved to get a break from Satan's prescription.

Chapter 18

Don't Keep Secrets from Your Friends

I was coming off being sick from the Nerlynx and preparing for the implant transfer for the month of December. It was decided that I would take eight weeks off to get the surgery and get comfortable with going back the Nerlynx. I needed to get to the point that I would not spend the entire day in the restroom. Dr. Laura and I had talked, and we needed to figure out a way to stop the diarrhea and would experiment with a combination of anti-diarrhea medicines. I was her first patient to ever take this type of target therapy, so everything was new to her as well.

I had appointments with Dr. Teddy, the plastic surgeon, and we were a go. I had the size implant chosen and was ready to get this done. It was also exciting that I would be getting my port taken out. Many people with ports keep them in since it was an easier way to do blood work, and sometimes a chemo patient burns out their veins, so a port is usually a necessity.

This was an outpatient surgery, so once it was over, I was headed home. It was planned again for early in the morning, but this time, TJ and I decided not to stay over at a hotel for the evening prior. We got up early, and I went through the usual routine of showering with the antibacterial soap. I packed pajamas to wear home. One thing about going through so much treatment and so many surgeries is that in the beginning, I would have been mortified to be seen out in my pajamas. Now I had no issue with coming home from the hospital in my jammies. If anyone looked at me funny, my response was "I have cancer." That always ended any questionable glances.

This surgery was no different than any of the others. I checked in and went to the same room as before. Another déjà vu moment, I know I have done this before. Dr. Teddy came in, happily asking how my Vegas vacation went and if I had my rock star moment. We went through all the procedures of the day, and I was ready to get it over with and move forward. I certainly would not miss the tissue expanders and was ready to welcome my new breast implants.

The surgery was uneventful. My sides were sore as Dr. Teddy had completed liposuction to do a fat transfer. He had filled in areas around the breast implants and where the port had stretched skin. Home I went and directly to bed. This was my usual routine. This time, I did not have the worry of dealing with drains. I think that Madison was secretly disappointed because she always took charge when I had drains.

As the days went on, the part of my body that hurt the most was not the breast area but the area of the fat transfer. I was black and blue up both my sides and along my front lower abdomen. Looking in the mirror, I looked like I was in a mixed martial arts fight and lost. The bruising was far worse than I had expected. Doing simple movements such as pulling myself to a sitting position from lying down was very painful. On a positive note, my new breasts looked great. I had minimal scaring from the original mastectomy, so with this new surgery, Dr. Teddy cut along the original lines. This way, he was not creating any new scars.

My first evening out was a girls' night with my friends Christy Ann and Karrie. It was our pre-Christmas celebration. Since I was not able to drive, Christy Ann came by the house to pick me up. I was moving a little slower than normal but was grateful to get out of the house. We didn't even make it out of the neighborhood, and she started on me. She had a lot of questions. *How are you doing? What is your treatment plan? Why were you in the emergency room? Why did I have to see a post about you not doing well on Facebook?*

Christy Ann was full of questions, but full of comments as well. Her last question stung a little. *Are you telling me the truth about your condition?* The truth was that I was never dishonest about what was going on, but more so omitting some of the important things. I had always been one to just tell everyone that all was going well. I think that deep down, I wasn't honest with myself as well as my friends. I knew that Christy Ann's inquisition was because she cared. She and Karrie were important people in my life, and I realized that it wasn't fair sugarcoating things to them. Karrie joined us at the restaurant, and it felt good to be with my friends. After an evening of laughing and me not needing to follow a BRAT diet, we started to leave. The three of us were in the restroom when I said, "Do you want to see my new implants?" Of course, they both wanted to see my plastic surgeon's work, so I lifted my shirt and the surgical bra up. Both of their eyes went directly to the liposuction bruising. I think that the sight of the breasts with no nipples and the liposuction bruising was a bit too much for them. It was probably more of a horror show for them. To me, it looked great compared with some of the women I had seen online going through this procedure. Maybe, Christy Ann and Karrie needed something to compare it with to be as impressed as I am. We agreed that we would get together for dinner before Christy Ann left town after Christmas. It was agreed that our next girl's night would be the day after Christmas. That was also the date that I was to start the Nerlynx again.

It was Christmas, and I may have shown people at the Christmas Eve dinner my new implants and scarring. I enjoyed the holidays but knew that I would be doing the target therapy again. Would I get sick again? I was going to take Imodium to help me not have diarrhea. I thought that it was all figured out. The day after Christmas arrived, and I was stalling the process of taking the Nerlynx . Four days prior, I had been taking Imodium to get it in my system. I finally took the Nerlynx and went to take a nap before my night out to dinner with Christy Ann and Karrie. I woke up two hours before dinner and felt terrible. I was nauseous. Then it started. I was vomiting, and I could not stop. It seemed that once I started vomiting, the diarrhea wasn't far behind. I had gotten some vomit on the floor, and when I went to clean it up, I noticed it had taken the finish off the floor. The thought crossed my mind that if I was putting this purposely into my body and it was doing this to my floor, what was it doing to my insides?

I was violently ill. It got to the point that it was not possible for me to leave the bathroom. I had texted Christy Ann and Karrie and said that I wasn't feeling well and could not make it to dinner. TJ was downstairs, and knowing that I had dinner plans, he came upstairs to see what I was up to. That was when he found me. I was lying on the bathroom floor. I didn't remember a lot from this time because I was a bit out of it. Once again, I was having fluid flying out of my body at both ends, and I could not stop it. I could hear TJ talking to someone. It was 911. Madison came upstairs and started to help pack a bag and gather my medications. It seemed as if the ambulance arrived immediately, or maybe I was too out of it to notice the length of time. Madison helped me change my pajamas because I had soiled myself.

I could hear the ambulance crew talking to TJ and Madison. They were telling the crew of my condition and the medications that I take. I could not make it down the stairs, so a special chair was brought in to take me down the stairs. Like I said, I don't remember much, but the things that I do remember have stuck with me. I remember being in the ambulance and the paramedic starting an IV. It seemed as though things were just mere flashes of time. I remember the stick of the IV and the bright lights of the ambulance. The worst was seeing my parents, my brother, and especially Morgan, who was standing in the driveway, watching with sadness. I wanted to tell Morgan that everything would be okay, but I wasn't sure myself if that were true. I remember the ride to the hospital. Facing the back of the ambulance and already having nausea, I remember wondering if I was nauseous from the medicine or the ambulance ride. The ride to the hospital seemed to take an eternity. I made a grand entrance to the emergency room with loud vomiting and heaving. I didn't care about anything but feeling better.

TJ and Madison followed the ambulance and waited for me in a room. They both looked frightened because this was the worst of any of my emergency visits. All my other visits to the ER I was confident that I would walk out with a solution to my problem. This time, I wasn't sure.

I knew that this time, it took longer to get things stable. In the past, I could make it to the ER with the help of TJ and not needing all that happened this time. This time was different. Lying in the hospital bed and hearing the commotion of the ER staff working around me and seeing TJ and Madison standing together in a corner with fear in their eyes was too much to handle.

It seemed as quickly as things happened, they also slowed down in that manner. When I was stable, that was when the pain hit. I was still recovering from a surgery, and the motion of nonstop heaving felt like I had been beaten with a sock full of nickels. I also had the bruises to look like it happened as well. One of the first things I asked the attending nurse was if I had damaged any of Dr. Teddy's work. I was just sure in my mind that I had ripped some stitches out somehow. Luckily, everything looked as if it survived this adventure. After hours of observation and debating on whether I should stay at the hospital or go home, I was released. I felt 100 percent better and wanted to do my recovery at home in my own bed. Dr. Laura had been called, and she said to stop the Nerlynx until we can discuss some things. I promised to complete the follow-up and rest so that I could be released into the wild again.

My start with Nerlynx was not good. In my mind, the big, scary thought of not taking this target therapy and my cancer returning was haunting me. I had to figure out a way to get this therapy completed without it killing me.

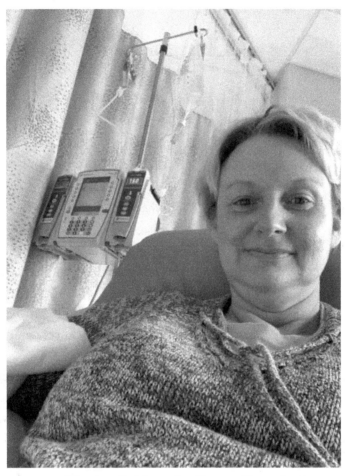

(Getting fluids at the Cancer Center)

Chapter 19

Roller Coaster

The next few months seemed like a roller-coaster ride that just would not stop. I followed up with Dr. Laura, and it was agreed that I would continue the target therapy of Nerlynx. If I could finish this year of therapy, my survival rate would increase. I needed those odds to work in my favor. Every time I would look at my family, it reminded me that I needed to stay steady on this course and make it through the therapy. I wanted to be with them through all the milestones like graduations, college, marriage, and families of their own. I wanted to grow old with TJ. I felt that if I couldn't do this therapy and the cancer came back, I would only have myself to blame.

The plan for me was to start the Nerlynx again once I recovered from my hospital trip. I would do one pill at a time for a week and progress until I hit the six pills again. This time, the difference was that I would take a prescription-level Imodium and anti-nausea medication. I dreaded the first day, but I took all the medication and waited. It didn't disappoint. Within minutes, I was throwing up and having diarrhea. It wasn't as dramatic as the previous times, but it still was not pleasant. It seemed that as soon as it started, the vomiting stopped. The diarrhea was still off and on during the day.

As the weeks progressed, the more pills I added to my daily routine. I had figured out the way to stop the vomiting, but the diarrhea was relentless. I was losing weight quickly, and that became a big concern to Dr. Laura. It was decided that I would come in once a week to receive fluids. The diarrhea was so frequent and fierce that I was dehydrating each week. Dr. Laura also wanted a panel of blood work completed to see just how well I was doing. One thing that was a trend was that I was always weak and tired. After looking at the blood work, Dr. Laura found that I was low in potassium. The normal range of potassium is 3.6 to 5.2 millimoles per liter (mmol/L). My potassium was hanging around in the low 2 range, which required urgent medical care. This was when I found out the dangers of low potassium. I learned that low potassium could cause muscle weakness, feeling cramped, and abnormal heart rhythms.

Each week, I went to the cancer center to receive fluid treatment and sometimes one to two bags of potassium. It was amazing how much better I would feel after getting the potassium back into my system. This called for a slow pump because potassium could burn as it went through the veins. When I had my port, it blocked that burn. Now that the port was gone, I was using a basic IV that was sometimes in my hand between the knuckles. This was painful without the flow of potassium, and it intensified with it.

As the weeks progressed, it became harder and harder to access a vein. I was limited since my cancer and my lymph node removal was on the left side and all vein access was required on the right side. I could see the stress the nurses were having, trying to access a vein. My arm looked more and more bruised with each visit. After a while, Dr. Laura decided it was time for the PICC line discussion. I had seen people with these before, and it looked like it was not an enjoyable experience. It actually looked rather intimidating and possibly painful. A PICC line is a catheter tube that is inserted into the neck, arm, or leg. The PICC line is positioned into a large vein that carries blood to the heart. Using this type of catheter is important for someone receiving long-term fluids. My mind was swimming. I was getting ready to go back to work, and I was not settled on the Nerlynx. There was no possible way that I could make it through a day in school. I would probably spend more time in the faculty restroom than teaching.

Sometimes, miracles come disguised as something not so miraculous. This time, something hit our world like an out-of-control meteor. It was called COVID-19. This illness changed everything that everyone knew. I had heard the rumblings of school closures and business lockdowns, but I was so absorbed in how I was going to get myself back into work mode that I may not have seen this coming as everyone else. The first thing that happened was that TJ's school division shut down. He worked over the state line in the neighboring state, so I was unsure if this would happen where I worked. I wanted to be prepared no matter what, so I got everything prepared for my return even though I had no clue how I would make this work. Things needed to be taken care of before returning. These included doctor appointments and even an oil change for my car. I knew that I would need to take time off to get fluid and potassium infusions each week. Taking time off would be limited. As I was sitting in the car dealership, waiting for my oil change to be complete, something happened that changed my whole return to work. As I was watching the dealership television, the regular programing was interrupted for a message from our state governor. The governor had decided to shut down schools for initially two weeks. This decision was to start the following Monday, which was the day I was to return to work. Even though I was shocked, part of me was secretly relieved because I was not sure how I was going to survive the return. The two weeks that was designated to assist in stopping the spread of COVID-19 turned into a three-month school closure. I returned to work in the virtual capacity, which was a small blessing for me in what turned our world into a roller-coaster ride of change.

I continued the entire spring on Nerlynx. This included going to the infusion center once a week to get fluids and potassium. The day finally arrived that I had no choice but to get a PICC line. My veins were begging for mercy, and there was no other choice. It was difficult to get scheduled at first. With the COVID-19 pandemic, getting any form of elective surgery was near impossible. Luckily, it was critical that I get this so that I would not have a worse health situation. I had seen people with these lines but knew that they were usually only temporary. I had no idea if I could make it the full year of this medication, but I had already made it through three months. An appointment for this procedure was quickly made, so I had very little time to build my anxiety of this.

I was told how easy this procedure would be, and because of COVID, I had to go by myself. Everything seemed to go as expected. The only pain was the injection of the local pain shot. But there was a problem that I did not expect. Because of COVID, I was required to wear a mask throughout the entire procedure, and part of the procedure was a paper covering that went over the patient's face. If I had issues with small spaces before this, it guaranteed an issue after wearing a mask and a sheet over my head. I was starting to sweat, and the paper covering was sticking to my face. It seemed as if it was a lifetime of lying there and watching a screen that showed the location of my veins. When it was over, I looked to see this intrusive piece of a medical device. It was placed between my elbow and shoulder on the inside of my right arm. It was impossible to hide. I quickly asked the nurses if there was anything that could cover it. I was afraid that it would draw attention and possibly gross people out when they notice it. I knew that once again I was dealing with a procedure that I could not get the area wet. Unfortunately, with the port, I had to wait for it to heal, but with this, it could never get wet. How would I shower? I couldn't go in the pool or go in the water at the beach. It seemed like the things that I enjoyed were definitely going to be restricted. The nurse said that she would get me a sleeve to cover it. What she returned with was what basically resembled a stretched-out tube sock that she slid over my PICC Line. My arm was so skinny that this "cover" fell down to my wrist. The nurse took some tape and positioned it back in place and taped it down. I was horrified. This was not what I had expected. Was this the best way to cover this line? I asked for suggestions on keeping the area dry and was given ideas, such as raising my arm out of the line of water in a shower and wrapping my arm in cling wrap with medical tape, sealing off both ends. How would I be able to maintain this for up to a year? It didn't seem possible or realistic.

Even though the PICC line was intrusive and annoying, it served a purpose. The next appointment at the cancer center proved its worth. I was connected to the fluids within minutes. There was no stress in trying to find a working vein because it was ready to go. It also helped with the potassium infusion. Normally, a potassium infusion going directly through an IV burns. It felt like someone lit my arm on fire as it pumped through my veins. An added plus of a PICC line or port is that the infusion of potassium is painless. This was a good thing for me since starting the Nerlynx made my potassium levels plummet. Each week, I heard the same news from the blood work. My potassium was getting lower and lower.

I had the PICC line for about five months. Through an internet search, I found a sleeve that delivered the right amount of coverage and compression. Also, I found a PICC line shower sleeve that resembled an arm floatie for kids. This was a tremendous help and allowed me to put my arm down and not worry about the area getting wet. I used both of these sleeves on a daily basis. Once the time for me to have the line came to an end, these PICC line fashions were in tatters and ready to be retired.

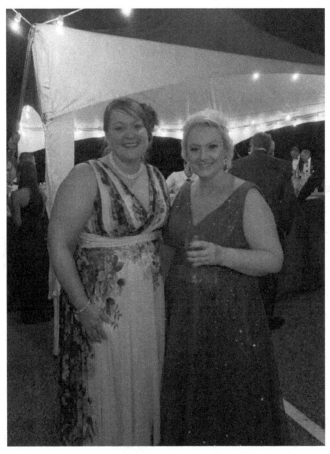

(Riverside Shore Memorial Hospital Ball
with fellow survivor, Stephanie)

Chapter 20

Stop This Ride, I Want to Get Off!

COVID-19 made a difficult situation even more difficult. I had several more emergency room situations over the summer months. These visits were even more challenging with all the restrictions. I had a visit that was TJ dropping me off at the front door and sitting in the parking lot to FaceTime me for updates.

As the days went by, I looked worse and worse each day. The dehydration and low potassium had a bad effect on my appearance. There were even rumors going around the community that I was at the end of my battle with cancer and nearing death. Yes, I knew my appearance was showing the strain. When I was working from home, teaching virtually, I would review the videos of me teaching a lesson and see that I definitely looked ill. In my mind, I was not losing this battle, but my appearance said differently.

I made it through the summer with the excitement of COVID and a PICC line. After hearing the near-death rumors, I tried to overcompensate by always making sure that I had my hair and makeup done. Unfortunately, all the makeup in the world did not make me look healthy.

I was so physically drained that it was a struggle to do normal things. The Nerlynx was causing uncontrollable diarrhea, and I was rapidly losing weight. At the end of my time taking Nerlynx, I had lost fifty pounds. I also started to have difficulty with randomly fainting. I tried to keep these instances to myself because I didn't want to alarm TJ or our daughters over this new side effect. Plus, TJ had seen me weak and sometimes a bit disoriented, so he had been threatening to revoke my driving. I found that there was only so long that I could keep this a secret.

My daughter Madison had asked for me to go with her to get our nails done. She drove, and I was thrilled to get out. I would, of course, have to wear a mask as my state had made it mandatory to wear a mask during this pandemic. We arrived at the nail salon, and I felt fine. Everything was going great. There were not many people in the salon, so we were seated almost immediately. The nail tech started to work on my nails, and I started to feel weak and sweaty. Madison looked at me and instantly noticed that something was not right.

"Mom, are you okay?" Madison asked. She could tell that I was not feeling normal.

I needed to put my head down. The nail tech went to get me a bottle of water and offered to get me a piece of cake. I assumed she thought that I was having a diabetic episode. The water was a blessing, but I felt so weak and needed to put my head down. I did not realize how much attention I had drawn in the salon. It came to a point that I had to put my head down on the salon table. The nail tech said she would stop doing my nails and asked Madison if she should call an ambulance. I could still hear what was being said around me, but it was muffled. I mustered enough to tell the nail tech to keep doing my nails and I would be all right in a few minutes. Nervously, the nail tech continued to file, buff, and paint my nails. I continued to keep my head down and prayed for this feeling to pass. The nail tech asked Madison again if she should call an ambulance. Madison addressed everyone in the salon, letting them know that I had cancer and had moments like this and to wait a few minutes to let it pass.

It took some time, but I did start to feel better, and luckily for me, my nails were done. The nail tech walked with me to the cash register and asked me over and over if I felt better. Then she was worried that I was going to drive. I reassured her that I would not be driving. Every time that I go to this salon, they automatically offer me water and a snack. I assume it is because having a passed-out woman at your nail salon is probably not good for business.

Madison proved to not be able to keep a secret because she immediately told TJ what had happened. He was upset with me and stated that he was "clipping my wings." I was officially restricted from driving. He even got my parents onboard with this, offering to drive me to appointments so I did not get an opportunity to drive myself.

My next fainting episode was again with Madison. She was starting to worry that every time I would go somewhere with her, I would get sick. This time, Madison wanted to get her ears pierced for the second time. Since she was under the age of eighteen, a parent must accompany her to get the piercing. Madison drove me to the mall so I can serve my role as parent, even though she seemed to be taking more care of me than vice versa. I felt fine for the moment. We were in the store where the piercing would take place, and it hit. My stomach was churning, and I was about to have diarrhea. I told Madison that I would be right back and needed to use the mall restroom. By the time I returned to the store, Madison was still waiting for her ear piercing because there was only one sales associate and a store full of people. I was standing around, waiting, and I started to feel faint. I did not want to draw attention like my visit to the nail salon. Trying to act upbeat, I said to Madison that I was going to sit down on the floor while we wait.

"Ewww, Mom, it's a dirty store floor. Why would you sit on the floor? You are not feeling okay, right?" Madison said.

I was caught. She knew that it was not normal for me to randomly sit on a store floor. I kept it together while Madison got her ears pierced. Then she had to go and pay the lady for the service, but there was already a line of people waiting to make their purchases. It seemed that everything was moving in slow motion. I moved myself off the store floor and into the piercing chair. I hoped that I would feel better, but I was sweating profusely, feeling weak and dizzy. It seemed like time was stopping. I leaned my head against the wall and braced myself so that I wouldn't fall out of the chair. Like the first time, it passed, but the whole ride home, Madison swore up and down that she was not taking me anywhere again. Also, as soon as we arrived home, she was quick to tell TJ every single detail.

Things were getting worse and worse, but I had stayed firm with taking the Nerlynx for nine months. I had a standing Wednesday appointment at the cancer center for fluids and potassium. One week in September, I felt the worst I had ever felt. I was weak, my whole body felt like it was cramped, and I was nauseous. By Tuesday, I could barely get out of bed without getting dizzy and needing to be back in bed. I feel that I have a strong faith even if I am not always in a church on Sunday mornings. I believe that sometimes a higher power comes into play to change the dynamic of a situation. On this Tuesday morning, I was debating if I should call the cancer center to see if they possibly had an opening in the infusion room. As I was lying there, trying to get the strength to call, my phone rang. It was one of the nurses from the infusion room letting me know that they had a cancelation and asking if I wanted to come in a day early for treatment. I was so grateful and agreed to be there within the next forty-five minutes. The challenge for me was how to get dressed when I have to lie down every five minutes. My mother was going to drive me to the cancer center, and because of COVID regulations, she would leave me, and TJ would pick me up on his way home from work.

The moment I staggered into the cancer center, the ladies at the front desk showed their worry for me. They made sure that I went back to the infusion room in a wheelchair because I was just too weak to walk back there. Once I was settled in the infusion recliner, one of the nurses, April, who was always no-nonsense, was quick to let me know that I did not look good. She was right. This was bad, but I didn't know at this time just how bad. April drew blood from the PICC line and sent it off to the lab to see just how bad things were this time. She hooked up the regular fluids but needed the result from the lab to determine how much potassium I needed.

When the result came in from the lab, April came back with a bag of potassium and a very serious look on her face.

"Are you having shortness of breath or chest pains?" she asked.

"Well, yes, I really just feel weak," I replied.

"It's not good. Your potassium is 1.9. That is critical, and I am letting Dr. Laura know so she can make a decision on what to do with you."

Critical was all I heard. I sat for two bags of potassium and waited for Dr. Laura to visit me and go over the lab work. TJ had a strong feeling about the Nerlynx medication. He wanted me off it. It had been a major issue of contention in our home life. He would tell me over and over that taking the Nerlynx was like committing suicide in slow motion. Each morning, before leaving for work, he would wake me up. I thought that it was because if he didn't get to sleep later, no one was allowed to, but he later shared that he woke me up before leaving because he wanted to make sure that I was still alive. It was his fear that our daughters would find me dead. It gave him a little hope that I was still alive when he left.

I, on the other hand, could not see his logic. My feeling was that if I stopped the Nerlynx and my cancer returned, I would only have myself to blame for not toughing it out for a full year. I was determined. My parents didn't raise a quitter.

Dr. Laura arrived at my little cubby area in the infusion lounge with a weary look on her face. TJ had texted me that he was in the parking lot of the cancer center and wanted to know what was going to happen. Because of COVID restrictions, I would just FaceTime him so that he could be a part of what was going to happen. I had packed my bag and had my purse on my shoulder ready to break free when Dr. Laura announced that since I was critical, I needed to stay the night at the hospital.

"Wait, what? An overnight stay at the hospital? I am not prepared for this," I exclaimed. "I need an overnight bag, my computer, and web camera. I have work to do."

TJ and Dr. Laura were quiet for a moment as we were all processing what needed to be done. TJ brought up the issue of whether I should continue with this medication. Dr. Laura made it clear that the continuation of this medicine was strictly up to me. She did not feel that it was ethical to sway me in any way to how I should continue. She also told us that just because I would complete a year did not a guarantee that I would be cancer-free. I wanted to know if my nine months of torture on this medicine counted for anything. Since it was a relatively new medication on the market, there was only limited data, but that data was positive. She advised that we talk about this tonight while I was captive at the hospital, and she indicated that she had another medication in mind, but it would take a longer duration of time to complete. I didn't feel completely hopeless. At least, there was a plan in mind if I decided to stop the medicine.

TJ left to go home and gather some personal items, and hopefully, by then, I would be in a room at the hospital. As I was being wheeled through the secret passageway from the cancer center to the main hospital, I felt defeated. I tried so hard to make it through the year, but my body was not accepting it. Nurse April wheeled me to the room that was waiting. She knew that I was down and was trying to be as upbeat as possible in this situation.

At the nurse's station, she stopped to let the nurses know that a "special VIP patient" had arrived. April had a good relationship with all the nurses there, and they greeted me warmly. As I was climbing into the hospital bed, April reminded me that this was a good decision. Another nurse joined us in the room. Her face looked familiar as she smiled and asked if I remembered her. I quickly looked at the name badge and realized that she was one of my fourth graders many years ago. My mind quickly hoped that I was a good teacher because now my former student would be giving me lifesaving medicine. She and April left, and I was suddenly by myself, pondering my next move. I had always been a planner, but this time, I didn't have a clue what my next move would be. I couldn't help myself and sat there and cried. TJ was busy on my overnight bag errand, and I didn't know whom to talk to. I texted my friends Christy Ann and Karrie. I had "gotten in trouble" by not keeping them in the loop. They were right; I needed to be open with them about what I was going through. They valued and cared about me, so it was only fair that I included them. I did it by text because they both were probably still at work. I immediately got a text back from Christy Ann, saying that she was glad to be kept in the loop and would call me shortly. She put in her text, "Thank you for holding up your end of the deal by telling us." She was right; I had tried to build this wall of everything was fine. The wall was definitely cracking. Karrie called shortly after and wanted an update. She told me that if I wanted to keep things personal, that was okay with her. I let her know that Christy Ann was right. I needed to be more open to the people closest to me. Karrie just wanted me to know that she was there for me and that she wanted me to be comfortable. We laughed about how we wouldn't tell Christy Ann that she was right and about how my nurse was my former fourth grader.

It wasn't long until TJ appeared with the list of things that I had requested for an overnight stay. He looked very stressed. We started to talk about what had happened, and I said that I was lost if I should stop the Nerlynx. This was a trigger to him. He became extremely upset with me.

"You have to stop. This medicine is killing you. It is like suicide in slow motion," he said.

He unloaded all his thoughts of what this medicine was doing to me. I just sat in the hospital bed with tears streaming down my face. TJ had enough. We were interrupted by a lady bringing a dinner tray. I had not eaten much and wanted to eat. TJ got up and walked to the door. He was going to go to the hospital cafeteria to get himself dinner, and he wanted me to think hard about what I was going to do.

I sat there wishing TJ was back in the room. I felt that this was a crossroads for me. I wanted to continue because of my fear of cancer coming back, but I also wanted to survive. He was right. This medicine was killing me. I knew what I needed to do. I needed to stop. All the big, scary what-if thoughts were in my head. Was I a failure for not finishing the time period of the medicine? I felt like a failure. TJ was gone for a long time, and I was worried that he was mad at me for considering the continuation of the Nerlynx. When he returned to the hospital room, he seemed to be in a better frame of mind. He had seen Dr. Laura in the hospital cafeteria. She went above and beyond her job by letting TJ vent about me and my stubbornness. She listened and told him that when it all came down to it, it was not her or TJ's decision but mine.

What they didn't know was that I had made a decision. The emergency hospital stay was the straw that broke the camel's back. I was afraid of dying. Mostly, my fear was dying of cancer, but now I was facing the possibility of dying from this medication. Dr. Laura had said that there were other options for medications. This was obviously not a good situation for me. I needed a change. I needed a change that would keep me alive. That night, I was hooked to heart monitors and received seven more bags of potassium. After all of that, I still did not reach the normal potassium number. I don't think I would have ended my relationship with Nerlynx if it weren't for this hospital stay.

Chapter 21

The Road to Healthy and Happy

As I reach the landmark of three years of my cancer diagnosis, I know that I will probably never be completely "out of the woods." Cancer will always be a part of my life. I let TJ know the night in the hospital that I was officially done with the Nerlynx treatment. Nine months of this should count for something. I was ready to feel healthy. Dr. Laura gave me some time to recuperate from the Nerlynx, and at the next appointment, we talked about the next plan of action for me. I would start a daily treatment pill of Tamoxifen. This medication would be a once-a-day pill that I would take for ten years. It was considered a SERM or a selective estrogen receptor modulator. It was one of the most prescribed and oldest medications on the market for women fighting breast cancer reoccurrence. Even though this medication was around for quite some time, its effectiveness was far less than Nerlynx. I had faced the reality that Nerlynx was not an option for me anymore, but I had the confidence that I made it through nine months, and that was better than nothing.

It took several weeks for me to come out of the Nerlynx fog. I was still experiencing a reduced level of the side effects as the Nerlynx worked its way out of my system. Luckily, those side effects were small compared with what I was originally experiencing, and there was no longer a need to receive weekly fluids. My potassium was now at a safe and healthy level. My energy level was building, and diarrhea was no longer a fifteen- to twenty-time-a-day experience. It was not even a daily experience.

Part of going through cancer treatment included making difficult decisions. Stopping Nerlynx was possibly the biggest decision I had ever made. It was a life-or-death decision. I admit that sometimes I think about what life would be like if I finished it. I especially thought about it on the day that I would have completed Nerlynx if I made it to the year mark. Yes, that was a tough day, but I also wondered if I had remained on the medicine, would I still be alive. I wondered if I had continued, how many emergency room visits would I have had.

Looking back, I know that I made the right decision. I had the PICC line removed and started to feel alive. Of course, I had to ask the typical questions when having the PICC line removed, such as "How bad will this hurt?" The nurse who was to remove it said that it would feel like a snake sliding out. That was not a helpful answer because my mind automatically wondered if it would be like a friendly green garden snake or a king cobra. The nurse told me to take a deep breath and then let it out slowly. While I was exhaling, she pulled the line from my arm. It was the little green garden snake that I had hoped for. After dressing the small exit area with a gauze pad and a bandage, I was on my way. I suddenly felt free.

I have been on Tamoxifen for several months and still have good days and bad days. The choice had to be made for myself to get off the roller coaster. Even though I wish I had a crystal ball to know the future of this story, I know that is not to be, and I will just have to embrace every twist and turn of life. Even in the toughest part of this journey, I was able to find joy and happiness at each moment, even the lowest. It is crucial for survival. If you take anything from hearing my journey, know that a positive attitude and strong positive people in your circle will keep you going and may even keep you alive.

Your Battle Is My Battle:

Cancer Caregiver

Thomas Johnson

Caregiver's Guide

I was inspired to share my story about my and my wife's journey with breast cancer. In March 2018, my wife discovered a lump under her left arm just under her armpit. We were walking our dogs on a windy day when the wind blew her jacket open. She reached over to pull her jacket and noticed the hard lump. When we arrived in the house, she told me about the lump and, of course, asked me to feel it. The skin was not red, and there was no sign of infection. It was just a quarter-sized, slightly elevated, hard lump.

This was the moment that our journey began. Since then, we have been riding an emotional and physical roller coaster. We have been through diagnosis, MRIs, chemotherapy, radiation, surgeries, plastic surgeries, hospitalizations, and recovery.

I hope that sharing my story as a cancer caregiver will help others through their journeys. Keep in mind that everyone's cancer story is different, but the lessons that I have learned can apply to anyone.

Listen

After my wife found the lump under her left arm, she was apprehensive about going to the doctor. She had every excuse in the world not to go. She told me, "It is probably nothing. I am going to have to take a day off during flu season." My wife is very hardheaded. She has an opinion or idea in her mind, and it can be very hard to move her off that stance. This is one of the things that I love about her but also one of the things that drives me crazy. I told her just go to the doctor.

Secretly, I think that she was also scared that it could be the worst of the worst news. After some complaining, she agreed and made an appointment. I was relieved that she did not stick to her guns and continue to hold out. I remember worrying about the situation and thinking about what this lump could possibly be. Could it be a cyst? My wife was forty-three years old. She couldn't possibly have cancer.

The weeks that followed consisted of more appointments and the dreaded diagnosis. When the doctor sat my wife and I down and gave us the news, it was like a ton of bricks landed on us both. Stage 3 breast cancer—how was this possible? This was where my journey started as a caregiver. As the doctor was explaining her diagnosis, I was observing my wife and her reaction. I knew that she was not processing this. I knew that she was in a state of denial. I knew that I needed to be the strong one. I was the one who was listening and really taking in what the doctor was saying because I knew she was not. I knew that her thoughts had gone to her children, to me, to her parents, and to the consequences of her situation.

During the first few weeks after her initial diagnosis, my wife flip-flopped in and out of a state of denial and what to do next. I cannot imagine the thoughts that go through someone's mind when faced with a potentially life-threatening disease. I know that it is very difficult to focus. My observations of my wife were surprising. To our family and friends, she was strong. She showed confidence and determination. She did not want to alarm anyone. She would say, "I am going to beat this. Don't worry." Privately, she was much more unsure of herself. She would ask me what would happen to our family if she were to pass. How would we survive? What effect would it have on our children?

Throughout all of this, I found myself doing a lot of listening. Listening to the doctors. Listening to my wife. Listening to my family and friends. My advice to any caregiver would be to do less talking and more listening, especially during the first few weeks. The shock of the situation will cause a lot of emotions that the people around you will need to express. They need someone to just listen.

Learn

If you have never cared for someone with cancer or known someone who has battled cancer, you have a lot to learn. Fortunately for me, I had never had someone close to me who was diagnosed with cancer until my wife's tragic news. I did not know what a stage 3 carcinoma was and did not know what kind of treatments to expect.

One thing that I did learn early, do not Google it. It will just get you down. Once you go down that path, you start to look up things like "stage 3 breast cancer life expectancy." This will only put your mind in a constant state of concern. It may be human nature that you would be concerned for your loved one's morality, but it is certainly not the route to take for your own sanity.

My advice is to use your time to learn about the little things that will help you and your partner through a difficult time. The best way to learn is to be present. Be present at your partner's appointments. Early on in this process, it was easy to be present. I had a job that was flexible, and I attended 90 percent of my wife's appointments. Listen to the nurses, medical professionals, and doctors. Ask them questions about your loved one's treatments, exams, and health.

Be present at home as well. It is easy to just try to forget about your problems and find a reason to be out of the house and not face them. That will be a huge mistake. Your loved one will have symptoms and side effects. You need to be there to learn what they need. Learn what they can and cannot eat. Learn what pills they need to take. Learn how much they need to rest.

I have learned more than I ever wanted to know about cancer. My wife has had forty doses of chemotherapy, twenty-five doses of radiation, four surgeries, and a nine-month prescription to the pill from hell. Chemotherapy was tough. They called the first few doses the red devil. The red devil was named because of its devastating effects. It makes you weak and makes your hair fall out. But there are other side effects as well. First of all, my wife's appetite and soda of choice changed dramatically. My wife and I used to eat a variety of foods, including weekly trips to Chinese and Mexican restaurants. After the red devil, my wife had to eat only the blandest of foods. They called it the BRAT diet, which consisted of bananas, rice, applesauce, and toast. Additionally, after the red devil, my wife became an iced tea and ginger ale drinker. Anything else, like soda, she said, just did not taste right.

As a caregiver, learn to take on new responsibilities. Treatment takes a lot out of you. My wife would sleep and rest some days for twenty out of twenty-four hours. Their body needs to recover, and rest is sometimes the best medicine. So being the parent of two daughters and keeper of the house became mostly my responsibility. I told some of my closest friends that, for about a year, I felt like a single father.

Radiation was not as bad as chemotherapy. There were not as many side effects. The biggest thing to remember was to keep the area well-hydrated with the cream that was prescribed. I remember that during radiation, my wife went back to work and was more of her old self at times. The day after she finished her last radiation, we even took a family trip to New York City. She was a real trooper. I remember being totally exhausted and looking at her and thinking, *How is she keeping up?*

I guess it is easy for me to say that the four surgeries were not too bad. I know that my wife was in pain, and again after each surgery, she got plenty of rest. The main thing that I learned is that I am not good with drains. If you have never experienced dealing with drains, let me tell you about them. Surgeons place drains in areas after surgery so that the area does not become infected. They are small tubes with a bulb that resembles a grenade. When the drains fill with blood, the drains have to be, well, drained. I am not one who does well with blood. I had passed out from getting a shot in the past. So I was not looking forward to draining the drains. Fortunately for me, my oldest daughter was interested in a future medical career, so she volunteered to do all the dirty work.

After all my wife's chemotherapies and radiations, the doctor prescribed her a pill that was supposed to reduce the chances of her cancer reoccurring, and that sounded great at first. I remember going to the appointment and hearing about this amazing new drug that would reduce the chance of her cancer coming back to the single digits. Wow, I thought this was great. Then came the side effects. The drug's side effect that hit my wife the hardest was diarrhea. This was not your normal diarrhea. This was ten-times-a-day crazy diarrhea. Over nine months, my wife visited the ER at least five times because of extreme dehydration. She lost over fifty pounds, and the "medication" put her potassium at dangerously low levels. When we were told that she was experiencing the signs and symptoms of potential cardiac arrest, we decided that enough was enough. This was an extremely hard decision for my wife. On one hand, she felt like taking this medicine may ensure her a longer life that was free of the worries of cancer returning. On the other hand, she was faced with potential cardiac arrest brought on by the very drug that was supposed to be our savior.

Accept help

When my wife first started treatments, people would say, "If you need anything, just let me know." I would always think that they were simply being polite and that most people were not sincere. Over time I found that I did need help and the people who really wanted to help just did things for us without asking if they could.

For example, our relatives would occasionally stop by just to take my daughters to dinner or shopping. For the girls, it was a welcome escape from our circumstances. It was also good to know that the girls were able to "get away" because my wife was in no condition to do all things that the family was used to doing.

Also, one of my wife's friends set up a meal train. This was organized online, and different people signed up to deliver dinners to our house most nights. It was really helpful, especially since I was working full-time and my wife was basically a full-time patient. Many of the people who brought meals were relatives, friends, and some acquaintances. Some of the people who stepped up to help out were people whom I would not have expected to do so. It was very touching, and I am and will continue to be grateful.

The biggest piece of advice that I can give is to ask for and accept help. This is a battle that is made easier by the people in your life who care about you and your family. When my wife was doing chemotherapy, I was working a full-time job, parenting two daughters, and being the caregiver for my wife, not to mention all the household duties that my wife and I used to share responsibility for. There is not a lot of downtime if you ever find yourself in a similar situation. So if someone wants to make your family a casserole, just let them. Enjoy not having to cook for a night. It is one less thing to do in an overwhelming schedule of tasks and duties.

Cheerlead

Throughout my whole experience as a caregiver, I was a cheerleader. A cancer patient needs one thing above all else—positivity. You have to be the one who says everything is going to be all right. You have to be the shoulder that your wife has to cry on. You have to be the one to say, "Yes, you are going to your treatment today."

It is not hard for someone to give up hope when in a situation like this. There were times when my wife would start to doubt herself. That is when you have to step in and be the positive voice that lifts them out of that space. There will be times when a cancer patient does not see the light at the end of tunnel. You have to be that light.

One time, I remember my wife getting very emotional and saying, "I have had enough. I do not want to go to treatment today." I replied, "I will be damned. You are not going to leave me with the kids and our parents. You are going to go to treatment and get better because I need you." She needed to hear that a lot of people in her life need her and that she needed to fight.

Do not get me wrong, these were just a few instances where my wife was feeling weak. For the most part, my wife's attitude during her sickness was very positive. She really changed as a person. Not that she was a bad person, but she definitely became more empathetic and caring for others in need. Others who were diagnosed with cancer instantly became friends with my wife. She would chat with them online and share tips about dieting, doctors, and treatments. We would find ourselves visiting individuals with care packages and stories to tell. These days, I cannot let her go into the local Walmart by herself because she will get into an hour-long conversation with someone about their cancer journeys.

Balance

It is so important to put things into perspective when your family goes through something like this. Make sure that you have your priorities in order. I was always someone with a job that carried a lot of responsibility. Luckily for me, my boss was very understanding and basically said, "Do what you have to do for your family as long as you get your work done." For me, it was easier to find balance. Balance between my work responsibilities and my family responsibilities. At the time, my family was much more important to me than any job could ever be.

Not everyone will have such an understanding boss. If you find yourself in this situation, take time off if you can. If a coworker can pick up some of the slack, let them. Do not expect to be able to go all out in your job. If you do, your family will suffer. Find the right balance for you between work and your family.

Give back

Eventually, things do slow down. My wife is now done with her major treatment. One of the things that we love to do is give back. This can be done in subtle ways and in big ways. Sharing our story and giving advice to other individuals who are going through this situation is very fulfilling. As I stated earlier, my wife has befriended several local individuals who have been diagnosed. Sometimes having someone to talk to who has been in your shoes is priceless.

My wife was also inspired to serve on the Ladies Auxiliary for our local hospital. They raise money for equipment and scholarships. We also find ourselves attending events for that to raise money for those in need much more frequently than before my wife's cancer.

No matter how you do it, volunteering, donating, or befriending, find a way to give back. It is always better to give than to receive.

CPSIA information can be obtained
at www.ICGtesting.com
Printed in the USA
BVHW030952100821
614084BV00009B/239/J

9 781664 178847